MW00679711

ALSO BY CHRISTOPHER NORWOOD

About Paterson: The Making and Unmaking
of an American City

At Highest Risk: Environmental Hazards
to Young and Unborn Children

HOW TO AVOID A CESAREAN SECTION

Christopher Norwood

SIMON AND SCHUSTER • NEW YORK

Published by Simon and Schuster
A Division of Simon & Schuster, Inc.
Simon & Schuster Building
Rockefeller Center
1230 Avenue of the Americas
New York, New York 10020
SIMON AND SCHUSTER and colophon are registered trademarks of
Simon & Schuster, Inc.
Designed by Eve Kirch
Manufactured in the United States of America

1 3 5 7 9 10 8 6 4 2

Library of Congress Cataloging in Publication Data

Norwood, Christopher.
How to avoid a cesarean section.
Includes index.
1. Cesarean section—Prevention. 2. Surgery,
Unnecessary—Prevention. I. Title.
RG761.N67   1984   618.8′6   83-20131

ISBN 0-671-46916-9

ACKNOWLEDGMENTS

The basic idea for this book began with a study of Cesarean section I did while working for the New York City Health and Hospitals Corporation. I would like to thank Frieda Nelson, Assistant Director of Health Statistics and Analysis, New York City Department of Health, for assistance in gathering statistics, and Dr. Jean Pakter, former Director of Maternity Services and Family Planning, New York City Department of Health, for reviewing drafts of that study and offering valuable advice.

I thank Dr. Harold Schulman and Theresa Dondero, midwife, for reviewing the manuscript and offering valuable advice and criticism.

For their support and assistance, I also sincerely thank my editor, Fred Hills; Martha Cochrane, Kate Connell, and Hilary Sares, editorial assistants; my agent, Virginia Barber, and her associate Mary Evans; and my typist, Audrey Ross.

And, I most appreciate the time and consideration which the many doctors, midwives, health educators and parents quoted in this book so generously gave me.

This book is dedicated to the accomplishments of the obstetrics departments of the New York City municipal hospital system (Health and Hospitals Corporation).

CONTENTS

7

———FOREWORD———

By HAROLD SCHULMAN, M.D.
Professor of Obstetrics and Gynecology,
Albert Einstein College of Medicine
and affiliated hospitals

D uring the past decade we have witnessed an important transition in the relationship of physicians to society. The post-World War II explosion of medical knowledge created a situation in which the doctor had an inordinate advantage over the patient. The physician was the recipient of new information in biochemistry, physiology and pharmacology, and the public was not. Hence the doctor-patient relationship became an encounter between an informed, usually authoritative person and a fearful, anxiety-ridden, poorly informed individual who was somewhat in awe of the other person. A number of forces during the past decade have served to correct this imbalance. Most important have been the media. Television, newspapers and magazines regularly inform the public, as well as physicians, of the latest advances and dangers in medical science and practice. The feminist movement has been extremely successful in pointing out deficiencies in man-woman relationships, and not unexpectedly has focused upon the obstetrician-gynecologist as a culprit.

This book is an excellent example of the movement to make the public as informed as possible about medical decision-making and medical problems. Childbirth is undeniably a social issue and deserves in-depth exploration by all sectors of society. On the issue of Cesarean section, there is clearly a problem. Whereas ten to fifteen years ago most physicians agreed that maintaining a Cesarean-section rate of 5 percent or less was important, today there seems to be no standard level of agreement.

Most recent surveys indicate a national average Cesarean-section rate of approximately 18 percent. As Chris Norwood points out in this book, there are disturbing differences among hospitals, communities and regions of the country. Some hospitals are doing almost twice as many Cesarean operations as the national average, while others are doing fewer. There seems to be no clear medical reason for these differences, so explanations need to be sought elsewhere. The most logical focus is the physician.

Physicians, although taught the scientific method, frequently do not make decisions based on probability. Ideally, when a medical problem is encountered, a controlled experiment should be carried out to determine which treatment results in the best outcome. The results represent the probabilities, that is, the likelihood that a given treatment will produce a given result. The reason that probability alone does not answer many questions is the element of risk. For example, if a woman has had a previous low transverse cervical Cesarean section, the probability of her uterus rupturing severely in the next pregnancy and labor is less than one in a thousand. However, a catastrophic rupture of the uterus endangers the life of both the mother and the baby. Thus many physicians decide that there will be less likelihood of a catastrophe if they perform an elective repeat Cesarean section, rather than allow labor. There is no disagreement about the odds, but there is dissent over whether the risk should be taken. Judgments regarding risk inevitably involve society as a whole. Chris Norwood takes the position that there are too many Cesarean sections being done, and that women should be better informed about this matter. I think that she is correct.

Medicine should never adopt the philosophy that surgery is superior to medical therapy. Physicians should strive to work with the body's functions, or use medications to encourage a return to a normal state. It is difficult to believe that we have evolved to the point where more than 20 percent of our offspring must be removed surgically in order to ensure good health for the mother and normality for the child. Chris Norwood's concerns are not those of an extremist, but those of an informed citizen trying to guide us back to a more reasoned approach to the problem of Cesarean section birth.

PREFACE

Within the past decade in the United States the process of giving birth has changed so drastically that, for the first time in history, almost one-fifth of mothers face the prospect that their babies will be delivered surgically by Cesarean section rather than by a normal, vaginal delivery. Clearly, for medical practitioners to change the birth process by which the human species has reproduced—and prospered—for eons is a major event; yet few mothers will find either obstetricians or birth educators who are willing to discuss this striking change with them. Nor would many parents be comforted to know that the side effects of Cesarean section, a major surgical procedure which alters the physiology of both mother and infant, have been studied less carefully than, say, the side effects of an over-the-counter drug like aspirin.

Although the death rate for mothers during Cesarean deliveries is well known to be two to four times that for normal births, only belatedly has research begun to focus on the impact on the babies; serious breathing difficulties, sometimes fatal, and anesthesia reactions may be more widespread than commonly supposed.

Still to be investigated at all is whether Cesareans pose a long-term threat to the physical, mental, or emotional development of a youngster. Under the circumstances, to subject mothers and babies capable of a normal delivery to the sometimes dangerous "fetal maturity" tests, major anesthesia exposures, intensive-care nurseries, and the depressing surgical atmosphere of a Cesarean birth is as senseless as subjecting a person in fine health to the rigors of cancer treatment.

With so much about childbirth having changed so quickly, and with new test procedures, new surgical "criteria," and new terminology coming into use at a pace that even doctors find daunting, parents may wonder how they can possibly learn strategies that will help ensure a normal birth for their baby. This book will present basic, straightforward information and practical steps which parents can use to reduce significantly the possibility of an unnecessary Cesarean.

As bewilderingly complex as obstetrics has become, the fact remains that 90 percent of mothers still have essentially normal, full-term pregnancies; to guard against unnecessary surgery, these mothers simply need to understand the few basic questions to ask when choosing a hospital or birth attendant. Mothers considered "high risk" may have to work harder and learn more to secure the possibility of normal delivery, but they will make few more rewarding efforts in life; for many so-called high-risk mothers, including those who have had a previous Cesarean and those with overdue babies, infant survival has actually improved at hospitals which have managed to reduce their Cesarean births. An abnormal delivery as the single-minded solution to an "abnormal" pregnancy is not always justified.

Learning about Cesareans, then, is not merely a convenience or a way for mothers to avoid the pain of surgery—although that is reason enough. In the current obstetrical climate, parents with a fundamental understanding of both the risks and the benefits of Cesareans have taken a major step to ensure the safe delivery of their baby and enhance the joy of birth.

Chapter One

THE CESAREAN
EXPLOSION

F or women who are pregnant now or expect to be within the next year, the chances are almost one in five that they will have a Cesarean section rather than give birth naturally. We have known for hundreds of years that, with rare exceptions, a vaginal delivery is infinitely safer for both mother and baby. Still, the incidence of surgical intervention in labor and delivery has increased markedly in the second half of this century, and *alarmingly* in the past decade. Growing evidence documents that over half of all Cesarean deliveries today are *not medically necessary.* Consider, too, something even more disturbing: despite sophisticated diagnostic technology, improved surgical techniques, and intensive-care nurseries, serious complications after Cesareans continue to haunt large numbers of both mothers and babies.

These facts give rise to a number of very important questions: Why have Cesareans become so common—even though they are less safe and often not necessary? How can a mother know whether she should have a Cesarean section, and which doctors and hospitals will cooperate with her if she wants to avoid having an operation?

Certainly there are times when a Cesarean section is essential to ensure the well-being of mother and child, and we will discuss those circumstances carefully. But mothers who want to guard against being swept up in the current fad favoring surgical deliveries will need to understand fully what a Cesarean section is, what the risks are, when it is the best course of action and when it is not. Parents should be aware of how this zeal for Cesareans began, and how to find a doctor who will be sensitive to their concerns and work closely with them to make the most intelligent decision about labor and delivery.

First, let's look at the operation itself.

What Is a Cesarean Section?

A Cesarean, while safer than many operations, is major surgery. The operation takes about an hour. The mother is anesthetized, her bladder drained with a catheter, and her skin scrubbed. After her abdomen is opened—more often now by a low "bikini" incision than a classical longitudinal one—her bladder is carefully peeled away from its position over the uterus and then the uterus itself is opened by incision, exposing the baby. With one hand under the fetal head and the other pressing against the uterus, the doctor guides out the newborn. The baby's removal usually takes between five and eight minutes. Its mouth is suctioned immediately with a small syringe to remove excess mucus from the throat. Oxygen may be needed to help the baby start breathing properly, and if there are breathing problems—which are rather common in Cesarean deliveries—it will immediately be sent to the nursery for observation and care as needed.

The placenta is removed after the baby, and then the mother stays for another three-quarters of an hour of careful repair. The bladder is sewn back into place, muscles realigned, and, in the end, there will be six or seven layers of stitches before the incision is closed. Most mothers spend four to six days in the hospital recovering, and many feel weak from the combined impact of anesthesia and surgical stress for weeks, or even months, after they go home. Complications, most commonly infections, occur in about half of all Cesarean deliveries.

The name "Cesarean" does not, as is sometimes assumed, derive from Julius Caesar's having been born by Cesarean section; we know that Caesar's mother lived until he was an adult, and the probability of her having survived such surgery in ancient Rome is about zero. More likely the name derives from Roman law, *lex caesarea,* which required that physicians cut open a mother dying in childbirth to try to remove the child. The first American Cesarean seems to have been performed in 1794 when Jesse Bennett, a doctor in Staunton, Vermont, operated on his own wife and, to general wonder, saved both mother and child. However, the high death rate—until the 1880s, the uterus was not sutured but left to "heal itself"—kept Cesareans from being anything except an emergency procedure. By the 1920s, improved surgical techniques made the operation somewhat more common, but severe blood loss and infection continued to be frightening hazards. Only in the post–World War II era, with blood banks to meet the high transfusion rate for Cesareans and with an array of antibiotics to fight the serious infection rate, has the operation been widely employed to head off potential or presumed problems, rather than for absolute emergencies.

Childbirth Is So Safe, Why Risk Surgery?

A most gratifying development of the twentieth century has been the extraordinary safety of childbirth. The chances of a mother dying in normal childbirth are now minuscule, and in industrial countries nearly all children who can possibly live on their own do survive the birth process. In the United States, even by the 1950s the chances of a child dying unexpectedly during a delivery when there had been a normal full-term pregnancy and no signs of trouble—in short, in the majority of deliveries—was very low, probably less than 1 in 25,000 births. Today, at most hospitals, the infant death rate for all deliveries, including the most difficult and high-risk ones, and the delivery of infants with severe malformations, is 1 or 2 in 1,000. With the sophisticated monitoring and testing now available to keep track of risky babies, many obstetricians predict that in the near future infant deaths during deliveries may be virtually eliminated.

The safety of Cesareans has also improved dramatically; fewer than 400 American women a year now die during childbirth. Still, Cesareans clearly are more dangerous. The death rate for mothers is two to four times that for vaginal delivery—and, some critics say, may well be twenty times higher, since the mode of delivery isn't always recorded on maternal death certificates. After surgery, mothers spend at least twice as much time in the hospital, and survey after survey has shown that about half experience serious medical complications, primarily infection. Transfusion of the mother is also required in about 10 percent of Cesarean births. Nearly all mothers report depression and general discomfort afterward. "The slowness of recovery often comes as a shock to Cesarean mothers, especially when they were talked into the operation as being the easy solution," comments Elizabeth Shearer, cofounder of C-Sec, Inc., a Massachusetts volunteer organization devoted to "humanizing" Cesarean birth.

After leaving the hospital, the mother may have persistent problems from wound abscesses, bowel or other organ perforations, and lingering bladder infections. The complication of Cesarean sections perhaps least mentioned by doctors, however, is hysterectomy following severe infection or hemorrhage. Recently, doctors at a large teaching hospital widely admired for the excellence of its obstetric surgery studied complications in mothers whose breech babies (breech infants descend into the birth canal with the feet and buttocks rather than the head coming first) were delivered by Cesarean. Two out of 148 mothers eventually underwent hysterectomy, thereby ending their ability to have children at all.

The babies, too, sometimes require special care for adverse effects. Respiratory distress, a disease in which the baby does not have adequate lung surfactant to breathe properly, is rare after vaginal deliveries, which "prime" the lungs to start breathing, but is a constant hazard of Cesareans; in severe cases, the babies are sent to intensive-care nurseries to be put on respirators and cannot go home for weeks or months. Neonatal jaundice, which may also require that the baby spend extra time in the hospital, although not as threatening as respiratory distress, is frequent among Cesarean babies. The fact that Cesarean babies who are sluggish from anesthesia sometimes cannot feed properly in their first few days of life can make jaundice more acute. And, as do mothers, babies sometimes sustain various surgical accidents, including cuts on their faces or other areas and unexplained infections.

Perhaps as important as what is known about the side effects of Cesareans is what is not known. If the post–World War II era has brought tremendous improvements in the ability of medical science to save abnormal pregnancies and sickly newborns, it has also taught, again and again, through tragedies like those of thalidomide, DES, and oxygen-induced blindness among newborns in intensive-care incubators, that the fetus and young infant are extremely vulnerable to permanent injury from misapplied medicine. Disturbing as it is in the face of these warnings, there has been no substantial long-term follow-up of Cesarean babies to determine whether surgical birth causes infant impairment which might only become obvious in later years. (Genital cancers caused by DES, for instance, usually develop fifteen to twenty years after the fetus is exposed to the drug by the mother's having taken it.) Any aftereffects of Cesareans would probably be subtler— for instance, slight biochemical malfunctions as a result of the infant's having been deprived of the intense enzyme surge and "priming" of its systems which occurs during vaginal birth, or nervous-system impairment from the anesthesia. What is certain, however, as medical practitioners continue to interfere blindly with the normal method of human birth, is that no one knows.

When Should a Cesarean Be Done?

Because any kind of surgery carries a number of hazards, Cesareans should be performed only to protect mothers and infants from death or possible harm. In a small number of well-recognized emergencies, including various problems with the placenta or umbilical cord, Cesareans are mandatory. (These are further discussed in Chapter 4.) There are also certain mothers, primarily those with diabetes or hypertension (discussed in Chapters 3 and 4), and babies, prominently breech infants (see later in this chapter and Chapter 3) and very large babies, for whom Cesareans may often —although not always—be preferable. In addition, labor can occasionally falter for other reasons.

There is almost no dispute that some increase in the very low Cesarean rates common a generation ago has

helped improved infant survival. For example, just
after World War II, a Scottish obstetrician observed
that when the Cesarean rate for first-time mothers in
Aberdeen changed from 1.1 percent to 3.8 percent of
deliveries, there were only half as many stillbirths.
However, today's Cesarean increases do not bring gratifying increases in infant survival. In fact, the National
Maternity Hospital in Dublin, Ireland, one of the few
large Western hospitals which has managed to stick to
a 5 percent Cesarean rate despite the Cesarean explosion, recently stunned the obstetric community by
pointing out that survival among babies born in their
hospital had improved faster than in the United States
with a Cesarean rate that has tripled in ten years.

But Aren't More Doctors Taking the "Natural" Approach Now?

It is interesting—and disturbing—that just when
parents are becoming so much better informed about
pregnancy, labor, and natural birth, the medical community has made so surprising a reversal in favor of
surgical birth. How did this happen?

In the early 1970s the childbirth education movement began to take root in the United States, and won
perhaps the most striking gain of all—freeing millions
of mothers from the apprehension and fear which have
historically shrouded birth. The movement has demonstrated that steps as simple as having a mother

change position or walk about can shorten the length of labor by hours; it has taught breathing and relaxation techniques which help control pain and encourage mothers to labor with as little medical intervention as possible.

But, at the same time, obstetrics was being inundated by a staggering range of new technologies—electronic fetal monitors, sonar, fetal scalp blood sample, estriol readings, contraction stress tests—all focused on the "risks" of pregnancy. The proper interpretation of these technologies and tests is still greatly disputed. A fetal monitor reading, for example, which one obstetrician uses to justify a Cesarean will earn only the contempt of the next obstetrician. Equally important, while parents were focusing on natural birth, these new diagnostic technologies threw the focus of obstetrics on the danger and pathology in pregnancy. The major result—a staggering increase in Cesareans—occurred, with no real research or analysis, almost overnight. "I can remember not many years ago," recounts Dr. Albert Haverkamp, chief of obstetrics at Denver General Hospital, one of the most respected public hospitals in the nation, "when the big topic at obstetrics conferences was how to get away from the obstetrics of terrifying women—you know, flattening them all with anesthesia and snatching the babies right away to the nursery—and move toward natural birth. But somehow, instead, we seem to have proceeded to the obstetrics of surgery and we simply have not paused to find out what we're really doing."

If the safety of childbirth is a high point of the twentieth century, the move toward unnecessary Cesareans

is among its tragedies. We now have all the necessary
ingredients for an obstetric and human triumph: well-
understood approaches to ease and encourage natural
labor and, standing by, sophisticated technologies
which can, *when needed,* help assure life for nearly all
babies. In theory, women today should enter childbirth
feeling a confidence both in themselves and in the
safety of birth which contradicts almost the entire
human experience of having children. Instead, most
women will find that hospitals are as clinical and cold
as they were before widespread childbirth education,
and also that, with technology focused on the hazards
of childbirth, medical attitudes have turned backward
almost to the thinking that shrouded childbirth in the
Middle Ages. Subjected to unnecessary tests, strapped
to machines, or shuffled off to the lab, mothers are constantly made to feel that labor is unpredictable, that
they can't do it themselves, and that what they need,
finally, is incisions, transfusions, stitches, and pain.

It is an atmosphere which can deflate the most joyous
expectations. Take the case of Esther Zorn, who gave
birth to her first baby in 1977 at a large teaching hospital with a 25 percent Cesarean rate, in Syracuse, New
York. There she encountered, almost step by step, the
typical textbook technology and interventions, horribly
divorced from human caring, that so routinely lead to
surgical birth. Ms. Zorn, now a founder of the Cesarean
Prevention Movement, had dutifully taken her Lamaze
classes, read instructional books—and then found herself in a world that seemed beyond comprehension.

"The birth began in the usual way," she recalls. "My
husband, Tom, was out parking the car and filling out

forms and I was left alone in a ward with three other women, who were all screaming. Already, I felt I was on an out-of-control assembly line. I quickly learned I hated enemas and intravenouses. I had many questions, but nobody had time to answer them. After seven hours of labor, my doctor came in and informed me that he was going out of town for a conference and wouldn't be there for the birth. Now, what he had done the day before was nick my membranes. [Nicking, or actually breaking, the membranes of the amniotic sac, which holds the fluid surrounding the fetus, can be done so simply during a routine vaginal examination—usually a small instrument is used, but a fingernail will suffice —that the mother may not even notice. The procedure starts labor artificially.] He, of course, knew that I would go into labor within hours—and he still did it planning to leave—but I didn't know that at the time. All I knew was that when he walked out of the room, my labor just stopped. They gave me sleeping medication against my will and then it was just a round of monitors, IVs, and Pitocin. [Pitocin, an artificial hormone, stimulates labor, but since it can put the fetus in distress, requires great care in its use.] I was petrified."

After thirty-six hours, Esther Zorn felt "terribly hungry" because she had not been allowed to eat, and generally awful because she had not been allowed out of bed, even to go to the bathroom. Like many people unaccustomed to hospitals, she was unable to use a bedpan. Finally, she was told she was going to have a Cesarean. In preparation for the operation, the nurses drained her urine mechanically with a catheter, and suddenly and surprisingly she became interested in pushing toward a vaginal delivery; up to this point, her distended bladder may well have been blocking labor. It is well recognized, although not always by hospitals, that women in labor should urinate once every hour or two to prevent a full bladder from impeding their progress. However, no one paid attention to her renewed enthusiasm.

"The next thing I knew," Ms. Zorn recalls, "I was numb from the spinal. As much as I remember it, the Cesarean was unpleasant, with a lot of grunting, tugging, pulling, and pain. Finally, they pulled Fred out. I reached out to touch him, but then I realized my hands were tied down. I wanted to talk, to say I wanted to touch him—they hadn't let my husband in for the Cesarean, else I think he could have interpreted for me —but my mouth was so dry from the anesthesia that when I tried to speak, no words formed. I started crying uncontrollably. The anesthesiologist looked down and asked me what was wrong, but I still couldn't speak. I remember he had such lovely blue eyes. And that was the birth. Today I realize how little I knew, despite the classes, about what can really happen—and what can be done to you—during birth."

Parents can crucially influence the way in which their child is born. But the time to start learning about choices—the reasons, the risks, the pros and cons of vaginal versus Cesarean childbirth—is not just before the birth, but before choosing a doctor or birth attendant, and a hospital. By the time a mother is in labor, and faced with a problem, it is dangerously late in the game to begin to ask questions.

An Alarming and Unstudied Explosion

Dr. Brooks Ranney, the 1982 president of the American College of Obstetricians and Gynecologists, has practiced for almost thirty years in Yankton, South Dakota, a service and shopping town, population now 16,000, for the surrounding wheat and oat farms. He is among the few American obstetricians who has gone through the Cesarean explosion without drastically increasing his own use of surgery. Reports from the lifetime records of his practice, published in the past few years, have been central to the reexamination of Cesarean practices in the United States. At the time Dr. Ranney stopped doing actual deliveries in 1977—he found, he explains, that after age sixty he could "no longer stay up all night to deliver a baby and then put in fourteen hours a day"—and limited himself to the prenatal care of patients, his Cesarean rate stood at 5.6 percent of the deliveries he performed; this is one-third the current national average. Having begun his obstetric practice right after World War II, however, Dr. Ranney also remembers when Cesarean rates were about 2 percent. "Looking back," he comments, "I can see some situations we could have saved by doing more Cesareans. Back then, we were perhaps too reluctant about the surgery.

"I would not like to say what someone else's Cesarean rate should be," he continues. "A lot depends on the health of the mothers you see, and the ones I see are pretty healthy. What does bother me is that, more and more, the reasons I hear for individual Cesareans are so vague. Any doctor who does a Cesarean has got to realize that he is changing something important about a woman forever—he is changing her childbearing. You don't just perform a Cesarean because of some squiggle on a machine. The doctor has got to have very good and specific reasons before he starts the incision. I am just not too thrilled when a resident says to me, 'Oh, I had to do a Cesarean. She failed to progress.' What does that mean? He hasn't told me *why* the mother failed to progress, and as far as I am concerned, that is too vague and the doctor has skipped a crucial step in his reasoning."

Because many Cesareans are performed for such vague reasons and because the rate has skyrocketed so quickly, there has been no opportunity to investigate, or really compare, the pros and cons of different birth methods for most mothers. If we know that Cesareans are beneficial in a small number of severe emergencies, or in cases of maternal or fetal illness, research has only recently focused on the possibility that high Cesarean rates may cost both maternal and infant lives. The mothers known as "repeat Cesareans" are a striking example of a group for whom surgical risks now apparently outweigh the risks of trying a vaginal delivery.

In the United States, ever since Cesareans became an accepted operation, obstetricians have assumed that another operation would be safer than attempting a vaginal delivery for Cesarean mothers who became pregnant again, even when the new pregnancy was perfectly normal. American doctors have lived by the dictum "Once a Cesarean, always a Cesarean," and some 98 percent of American women with Cesareans automatically have operations for the next delivery. By contrast, most European, and a few groundbreaking American, hospitals encourage previous Cesarean mothers to have a "trial labor" if their pregnancy seems normal and they have a well-healed, small "bikini" scar. We know that at least half of previous Cesarean mothers can deliver babies without surgery; recent research comparing twenty years of reports on trial labor in Europe and the United States—involving, all told, hundreds of thousands of births—showed some stunning results. The overall death rate for mothers who had repeat Cesareans was 1.2 times higher than for those who attempted normal labor; for babies, deaths directly related to the delivery were *three times higher for automatic Cesareans.* Evidently, the assumption that repeat Cesareans were safe was an error which had cost maternal and newborn lives by the hundreds for decades.

If this is the case for automatic repeat Cesareans, what about Cesareans performed for other reasons? Most Cesareans today are not even performed on mothers who fall into clear risk categories which might be claimed to justify the operation; they are performed on healthy women who reach the end of a normal, term pregnancy with a normal-weight fetus. Before being suddenly wheeled to the operating room, the mothers have had little if any indication that the pregnancy was so abnormal as to require surgery. For these mothers, the argument for the present Cesarean rate is disturbingly weak: for "primary," or first, Cesareans, except to some degree when the operation is used to avoid a difficult forceps delivery, infant survival does not improve.

Equally disturbing, rate increases do not reflect medical knowledge about which mothers may most benefit from a Cesarean. Older mothers—usually defined as women over age thirty-five—have about twice as many breech babies as younger women, and these babies are sometimes difficult candidates for a vaginal delivery. Older mothers may also be prone to "dysfunctional," or abnormal, labor—although evidently one important reason for this is that doctors, nervous about older women in labor, overmedicate them, and the drugs, in fact, halt the birth, necessitating a Cesarean. Yet, even if there is a medical basis for moderately higher Cesarean rates among older mothers, the rate for *younger* mothers has actually increased the fastest! Between 1963 and 1972, the Cesarean rate for older women in New York State increased by one-third, while it doubled for younger mothers; in California between 1960 and 1975, the Cesarean rate for women over age thirty doubled "and yet tripled for women under age twenty and for those aged 20–24 years, the latter a prime childbearing age at which complications tend to be minimal," a Department of Health, Education and Welfare study noted.

But the sharpest indictment of Cesareans is simply that some hospitals and individual obstetricians across the United States have, against the tide, maintained strikingly low Cesarean rates while at the same time achieving impressively good infant survival. There is nothing mysterious about what these doctors and hospitals do: they practice good obstetrics. They have deliberate strategies to prevent unnecessary Cesareans from being performed on normal mothers; and some have also initiated such well-conceived programs of care for "abnormal" mothers that they obtain close to normal survival for an array of difficult babies—breech babies, the babies of diabetic mothers, and postmature babies (those not born by the forty-second week of the pregnancy)—without resorting to excess Cesareans.

Los Angeles Women's Hospital, a public teaching hospital, has a seemingly impossible task; the largest obstetric hospital in the United States, it delivers some 15,000 babies a year, many the high-risk infants of teenage, poor, and malnourished women. Yet the Cesarean rate at Women's Hospital has been one-third below the national average for years. The hospital has steadily reduced infant mortality. Its clinical programs, from the midwife-run "Normal Birth Center" for low-risk mothers to its Postdate Clinic for overdue babies, are nationally admired.

As of 1980 North Central Bronx Hospital was the only hospital left in New York City with a Cesarean rate below 10 percent of births; yet infant mortality was lower there than at a multitude of New York hospitals serving healthier mothers.

Denver General Hospital has not just stabilized, but cut its Cesarean rate from 13 percent of births in 1979 to 10.2 percent in 1981; during that time, fetal and early infant deaths fell by 18 percent. "Don't get me wrong," Dr. Haverkamp, the chief of obstetrics, comments.

"When a Cesarean is really needed, I am absolutely grateful that the option exists. But with our population, which has the usual problems of a high-risk urban population, I don't think we could have done this if even a 10 percent Cesarean rate really contributed to infant survival. You just wouldn't expect that we could bring down the rate and the deaths at the same time. But we did."

In 1980, a highly concerned National Institutes of Health called a three-day conference on Cesareans, which was attended by experts across the nation. After examining survival statistics and other data for millions of American births, in an almost unprecedented policy statement about birth practices they concluded that the rise in Cesareans could be "stopped, and perhaps reversed" without jeopardizing the health of mothers or infants. To the contrary, these prominent obstetricians, midwives, and birth educators thought that *improvements* in both maternal and infant well-being could be made even if the Cesarean increase were brought to a halt; nonetheless, between 1980 and 1981, 150,000 more Cesareans were performed in the United States, and by 1982, 18 percent, or nearly one out of five, babies continued to be born by surgery. "Of course these figures are very discouraging," comments Ruth Lubic, a midwife who is director of the Maternity Center Association, for half a century a leading childbirth education center in New York City. "But I don't think the Cesarean situation will actually change very much until parents themselves begin to ask questions and insist on getting answers. On one level, it's not fair to put the burden on parents. Health professionals should figure out what they're doing. But, realistically, with the Cesarean rate what it is, all prospective parents should educate themselves about it. They can't assume this won't happen to them."

What Caused the Explosion?

Two recent reports which investigate the reasons for the Cesarean explosion will give parents a better understanding whether a Cesarean for their own baby is perhaps justified—or has been proposed for a reason that many experts consider inadequate. One report, "An Evaluation of Cesarean Section in the United States," was prepared for the Department of Health, Education and Welfare by Dr. Helen Marieskind, a public health specialist. The other, issued by the 1980 National Institutes of Health Consensus Conference, summarizes the general thinking of obstetricians, midwives, and public health specialists from across the country. While these reports do not agree in all their conclusions, they do concur that the causes of the Cesarean explosion are not simply medical—that is, having only to do with the baby's or mother's condition. Other factors, such as malpractice pressures, the difficulty of using new technologies, and the ways physicians are trained, have also exacerbated this disturbing trend.

Malpractice

Dr. Marieskind concluded that the threat of malpractice is now a major—if not *the* major—reason for the continuing increase in Cesarean deliveries. The hundred obstetricians she interviewed cited. fear of malpractice suits—obstetricians today are sued ten times more often than other doctors—as having both subtly and overtly discouraged them from proceeding with normal deliveries; if there was the slightest problem, a Cesarean could at least protect the doctor from the accusation of not having tried other measures. The new diagnostic technology reinforces these fears. Doctors feel that even though many test results can be misleading, any test readings that seem to deviate from "normal" can be used against them in court. "I don't think anyone can understand the Cesarean situation without spending some time in a malpractice courtroom," says the chief of obstetrics at a Chicago hospital. "If there's anything wrong with a baby, even when surgery would have made no difference, the first question is always, 'Why didn't you do a Cesarean?' If you did a Cesarean, the next question is, 'Why didn't you do it sooner?' "

Yet it is hard to tell precisely how often malpractice pressure is the deciding factor for an individual Cesarean. With all the variables involved in the decision, probably even the most candid doctors could not always say when they are practicing "defensive medicine." (Also, the Cesarean rate has risen in several

countries where malpractice suits are rare.) Nonetheless, doctors are willing to admit that legal considerations often win over sensible medical reasoning. The
chief of obstetrics at Cornell University Medical College in New York told Dr. Marieskind that despite the
great success of their policy of encouraging trial labor
throughout the 1950s and 1960s, by the late 1970s most
attending physicians refused to let previous Cesarean
mothers attempt normal labor at all; they feared that
this "departure from standard obstetrical practice"
could open them to legal suits. And, at a recent obstetrics symposium in California—the state where doctors
are sued most often—several doctors said that no matter what the evidence favoring vaginal deliveries for
some breech babies, in the current legal climate they
would continue to recommend Cesareans for every
breech delivery.

One way to get a rough idea of the overall role of the
malpractice threat is to compare Cesarean rates at private and public hospitals. Doctors at public hospitals
are protected from malpractice pressures because the
government provides their insurance protection and
because most of their patients have not yet developed
the middle-class tendency to sue at every turn. In New
York City, for example, by 1980, the Cesarean rate for
the city's public hospital system, which has twelve hospitals that deliver babies, had been stabilized at 15 percent for years; the average rate for the city's private
hospitals, on the other hand, had climbed continuously
to reach 20 percent of births by 1980. Doctors in the
public system often say "you can actually feel a release
from legal tension." Obstetricians at Army hospitals,

whose malpractice protection is supplied by the federal government, also cite their freedom from the pressures of defensive medicine in explaining their often low Cesarean rates.

Obviously, fear of malpractice is not a valid reason to perform any operation. But it does no good to blame doctors and hospitals alone for this; the American malpractice imbroglio is not duplicated anywhere else in the world, and it won't go away until the society as a whole comes to terms with it. Until that happens, parents must be aware that one important reason for the Cesarean increase is, absolutely and inarguably, not a medical one.

Automatic Repeat Cesareans: Outdated and Costly

In the United States, where "once a Cesarean, always a Cesarean" has been the rule, every increase in first, or primary, Cesareans has also meant a huge increase in Cesareans for subsequent births. Perhaps the most depressing thought for women recovering from a first Cesarean—whether they feel the operation was necessary or not—is that, if they want another child, they won't have any choice at all next time. "I think I began planning how to get out of this with my second before the anesthesia even wore off," one first-time Cesarean mother remembers. "It became the obsession of my life."

Repeat operations account for one-third of American Cesareans—200,000 a year. What is most amazing in this day of electronic obstetrics is that the policy of repeats originated more than fifty years ago. For early Cesarean operations, long vertical incisions of the mother's abdomen and uterus, which left large scars, were standard. Under the pressure of normal labor, about 5 percent of these uterine scars would rupture, creating a severe emergency for both mother and infant as bleeding and shock set in. At the time, then, it seemed the wisest course for Cesarean mothers to avoid labor entirely. Doctors began scheduling them for the operation toward the end of the pregnancy, even before their contractions started.

But, as early as the 1920s, doctors began to use the lower abdominal "bikini" incision. The bikini scar, which is standard today, so rarely ruptures that several large hospitals in Europe and the United States have seen literally thousands of "bikini" mothers through normal labor without a single rupture occurring. When the rare rupture does happen, while still an emergency, it is not usually life-threatening. In fact, there is apparently *not a single recorded case anywhere of any mother dying* when a low uterine scar ruptured; and, with modern care, the survival for babies is also approaching 100 percent.

This success with normal labor notwithstanding, most American doctors felt bound to automatic Cesarean repeats because this was the policy of the American College of Obstetricians and Gynecologists. The Consensus Conference urged doctors to attempt trial labor for appropriate mothers in 1980; finally, in 1982, and 400,000 automatic repeat operations later, the college, with some reservations, approved trial labor.

However, most obstetricians were not trained to handle trial labor and haven't been willing to make the necessary changes in their own procedures. So, automatic repeats remain the most frequent reason for unnecessary Cesareans.

Dystocia and Fetal Distress: Enter the Monitor

During the 1970s the number of Cesareans performed for dystocia, or "abnormal" labor, jumped by 30 percent to a total of 200,000 operations a year; fetal distress, a diagnosis based on interpreting changes in the baby's heartbeat, accounted for 5 percent of Cesareans. Since these are the two most frequent reasons why mothers who have had a perfectly healthy pregnancy end up with a sudden, unexpected Cesarean, it is especially important to understand dystocia and fetal distress. Unquestionably, both are overdiagnosed. Doctors write in medical journals again and again that, at most, there should be only one or two fetal distress Cesareans for every one hundred deliveries; and no one believes that in the 1970s hundreds of thousands of American women suddenly became unable to have normal labor.

Dystocia, the most common diagnosis for first-time Cesareans, involves problems of both anatomy and the quality of labor. Fetopelvic disproportion, in which a baby is too large to pass easily through the mother's pelvis, is the one dystocia diagnosis that is actually based on anatomy. And, because it does deal with physical dimensions, it is probably diagnosed the most

accurately. Even so, the diagnosis of fetopelvic disproportion attracts a certain controversy. There is a growing feeling in obstetrics that X rays, used for decades to
determine fetal–pelvic disproportion, expose the fetus
to unnecessary radiation while being unreliable as a
predictive tool. The skull is the largest part of the baby;
X rays may show the relative size of the skull and the
mother's pelvis, but, most of the time, they cannot predict what will happen during labor. Fetal skull bones
are still soft and pliable compared with an adult's and
may mold considerably to fit the pelvis, or the mother
may have a good, strong labor which will overcome
expected problems.

Perhaps the most forceful evaluation of X rays took
place a few years ago at Illinois Masonic Medical Center in Chicago. Illinois Masonic decided to halt all
X rays for its clinic mothers. As doctors began to evaluate cases individually rather than depending on the
presumed "predictions" of X rays, the primary Cesarean rate dropped from 10 percent of births to 8.9 percent. More important, this change of procedure forced
Illinois Masonic into the stunned realization that infant
mortality for clinic patients was actually lower than for
private patients—whose primary Cesarean rate stood
at 17.6 percent and still depended in part on X-ray evaluations!

With X rays in dispute, obstetricians have looked for
other means, including fetal weight and sonograms,
sound-wave measurements of the fetal head, to predict
disproportion. Yet, except for rare cases—an extremely
large baby or a major structural abnormality of the
mother's reproductive anatomy—disproportion still

cannot be predicted. Mothers who are told before labor
starts that the baby "won't fit" should question the doctor carefully. In nearly all cases, the doctor can be sure
that the mother has true disproportion only after a reasonable period of labor.

But anatomical disproportion does not account for
the entire 30 percent increase in "dystocia" Cesareans;
there has been an extraordinary leap in the diagnosis
of "abnormal labor"—a condition referred to by various vague and imprecise terms such as "dysfunctional
labor" or "dystocic labor" or "failure to progress."
There are two problems with Cesareans for abnormal
labor. The first is that the survival rate for babies of
normal weight—meaning 90 percent of infants—does
not improve. The second is that there is no general
understanding in obstetrics of when labor is really abnormal. Some obstetricians will say labor has "failed to
progress" after a certain amount of time has elapsed—
whether they, personally, choose to define that time as
eight, twelve, sixteen, or twenty-four hours. Other doctors might base their diagnosis on labor "slowing" at
some point, no matter that the mother is proceeding
within a normal time frame overall. Others seem to
throw in dystocia when they have no specific diagnosis,
but "feel" something is wrong with the labor.

Not surprisingly, the Consensus Conference said
there was "compelling reason" for doctors to start re-
thinking why and how dystocia is diagnosed. Virtually
all childbirth experts routinely answer "dystocia"
when asked to name the category of Cesarean births
they consider most unsettling. To Dr. Edward Quilligan, the chief of obstetrics who saw Los Angeles Wom-

en's Hospital through the general Cesarean surge, it is "the hardest diagnosis for a Cesarean to quantify." To Carol Hagin, a well-known nurse-midwife who practices in Walnut Creek, California, " 'Failure to progress' is the major reason for unnecessary primary Cesareans. In real fetopelvic disproportion, the body closes back up again. It's unmistakable."

"When you see the doubling and tripling of Cesareans for 'failure to progress' across the country, you just have to say that something cockamamie is going on in the way obstetrics is being practiced," says Dr. Haverkamp.

The increase in dystocia Cesareans raises a difficult question: Is dysfunctional labor simply being overdiagnosed (occasionally, labor does stop for mysterious reasons), or has obstetrics changed in ways that cause more women to have slow, weak labors? If obstetric practices do cause abnormal labor, mothers can learn to protect themselves from hospital intrusions which may impede the progress of the baby's birth. Childbirth is so intensely a psychological experience that the atmosphere created by a doctor and hospital is crucial.

To many critics—as to many mothers—the present atmosphere of hospital obstetrics departments, with their frantic efficiency, their beepers and buzzers and machines, seems almost certain to destroy the calm and confidence so needed during birth. Fetal monitors are the central piece in this drama. They measure fetal heartbeat patterns, either externally with a belt strapped around the mother's abdomen, or internally with an electrode inserted up the mother's vagina and attached to the baby's scalp. Because of continuing difficulties in interpreting the heartbeat patterns, nearly all hospitals seem to diagnose more "distressed" babies when they use monitors. This has been a problem since monitors came into wide use in the early 1970s. Only a few critics, however, have focused on the intriguing question of whether monitors increase dystocia Cesareans.

At Denver General Hospital, doctors began to wonder whether monitors sometimes "cause" dystocia. They were trying to determine whether basing Cesarean decisions on monitor readouts helped improve the immediate condition of babies at birth. So they divided 690 mothers into three groups: those to be monitored electronically during labor, those monitored electronically with the addition of fetal scalp sampling (a test used to show whether the fetus is getting enough oxygen), and those whose labor would be monitored the old-fashioned way, by stethoscope.

The electronically monitored group, the Denver doctors reported in *The American Journal of Obstetrics and Gynecology,* had the highest Cesarean rate—18 percent. With the addition of scalp sampling, the Cesarean rate fell to 12 percent, and with stethoscopes alone, was reduced to 6 percent. The doctors then thoroughly tested the physical and mental well-being of the newborns; they found no differences among the groups, so the tripled Cesarean rate for the monitored group apparently provided no benefits for the babies. There was another disconcerting result: When the doctors studied the birth records of the mothers, they found, as might have been expected, that most of the babies being delivered by Cesarean for presumed "distress" had been monitored electronically. What hadn't been expected was that monitored mothers also ended up with twice as many Cesareans for disproportion and "failure to progress."

"Surprised? You bet we were surprised!" comments Dr. Haverkamp. "Here we have the same doctors and nurses taking care of these mothers and making decisions about surgery—and, of course, the mothers in the groups were basically the same in terms of risk and age, and so forth. There were no medical differences between the groups at the start to account for the Cesarean differences. So, the only differential is the monitor. We've thought and thought how monitorings could double Cesareans for dystocia. After all, such Cesareans have zoomed everywhere; the Denver study only mirrors what has happened across the country. One conclusion simply is that, physiologically, the monitor impedes labor because it enforces lying on the back, and we all know labor goes better when the mothers move around and walk. But, second, I think monitors make many mothers nervous and tense. They're sitting there asking themselves, 'If labor is so safe and my baby's doing so great, then why are both of us hooked to these wires?' The doctors are also anxious. Before you had that machine in front of you, nobody sweated letting things go just a little longer, but now they're scared. The monitors were supposed to reassure patients and doctors. I think they may do just the opposite. It's not, of course, that mothers don't have to be monitored during labor, but there are other ways of doing it—for instance, a nurse with a stethoscope."

Another way of looking at this problem is to see what

happens when hospitals decide to *stop* using monitors for mothers who have had normal pregnancies. A few years ago the University of California at Davis Medical Center in Sacramento set up an alternative birth room where low-risk mothers were spared most standard procedures of "medical birth," including routine enemas, intravenouses, and being shaved. Especially, they were not monitored. "All concerned strove to achieve tranquility," Dr. Robert Goodlin wrote in the British medical journal *Lancet*. "Routine electronic fetal monitoring was considered counterproductive."

The primary Cesarean rate for mothers who delivered in this tranquil, nonelectronic atmosphere was 2.8 percent. Just doors away at the same hospital, low-risk mothers who delivered in standard, fully equipped delivery rooms had a primary Cesarean rate of 9.2 percent! The condition of the unmonitored babies was excellent. Their rates of distress at birth and of newborn jaundice were far below that accepted as "average" in American hospitals.

Let's also look more closely at fetal distress, the diagnosis which accounts for 5 percent of Cesareans. The majority of hospitals have simply never corrected the huge increases in Cesareans for fetal distress which accompanied the introduction of routine monitoring. Not only is there still difficulty—and incompetence— in interpreting monitors, but by providing a permanent record of the birth, monitors increase the legal pressure on doctors. The obstetrician may fear that monitor readouts with even small, meaningless deviations from "average" could be used against him or her in court.

In the present climate, hospitals with a 1 percent rate of Cesareans for fetal distress are considered to be doing very well indeed; yet there is no evidence that even that 1 percent is necessary. Doctors at the School of Medicine at the University of California at Davis, known for its "good" 1 percent rate of distress Cesareans, recently reviewed the Apgar scores of a large group of babies who, according to monitor readings, were in distress during labor. (The Apgar score, measured on a scale from one to ten, is a quick, standard assessment of an infant's appearance, alertness, and reflexes right after birth.) Half the babies at Davis were delivered by Cesarean, half not; either way, most of the presumably distressed infants had good to superior Apgar scores, and scores were slightly better for those delivered vaginally. The doctors concluded that "an [electronic tracing] classically thought to indicate fetal distress was wrong about 75 percent of the time."

The great tragedy of unnecessary Cesareans for misdiagnosed distress is that half or more of them could easily be prevented by a two-minute test. This fast procedure, fetal scalp-blood sampling, is simple, reliable, and painless to the mother. A small scalpel is inserted up the vagina and a few drops of blood taken from the baby's scalp. The blood is then quickly tested for acidity, a biochemical sign of distress. While it may seem unkind to greet babies into the world with a knife prick, the procedure has few side effects—only rarely do babies develop scalp infections—and sampling obviously is preferable to a needless operation. By showing whether fetal blood chemistry has changed, it helps doctors determine whether monitoring patterns which look "stressful" on the graph are just showing the acceptable, even necessary stress which occurs as the baby mobilizes to be born, or whether the baby is truly faltering.

For at least five years, clinical studies have demonstrated that scalp sampling could help avoid at least half the Cesareans performed when monitors are wrongly thought to signal fetal distress. Nonetheless, scalp sampling is used infrequently. In New York City, where because of the concentration of medical schools new techniques are used more readily than elsewhere, only seventeen of the city's fifty-five hospitals with obstetrics departments used sampling for at least 1 percent of births in 1980; the situation in other communities is more disheartening.

The words "Your labor is abnormal" or "Your baby is in distress" are naturally frightening to mothers. But before they accept such a diagnosis, mothers should keep in mind that the high Cesarean rate has not generally improved infant survival for dysfunctional labor and that distress is a hugely misdiagnosed condition of labor. There will almost always be time to ask questions and try other measures to improve the labor.

In both cases, if the mother has been kept flat in bed and immobile in order to use a monitor, what might help immediately is for her to change position, and especially to walk. When she is flat on her back, the force of gravity works against labor, and the uterus presses on the vena cava, a main blood vessel, decreasing the blood supply, and therefore the amount of oxygen, that eventually reaches the fetus. As a result, this position alone can cause fetal distress. If drugs have slowed the labor—they often do—wouldn't it be better for the mother just to rest and let the drugs wear off rather than proceeding right to a Cesarean? Did the baby's heartbeat take a sudden, serious drop, indicating an emergency—or, more commonly, were there only small changes in the heartbeat which might be quite natural and soon correct themselves?

What about natural means of encouraging labor?* A nice, long, warm shower has put many labors back on track. (Put a stool in the shower and sit under the water for a while.) Has the mother urinated often enough to keep her bladder from interfering with labor?

The wonderful aspect of natural labor is that it is not just a way to be born, but a way that prepares the baby to start breathing and functioning well right at birth. During labor, the baby experiences an enzyme surge that alerts its biochemical systems to the imminent birth; the stress of passing through the birth canal pushes out mucus and fluids from the respiratory passages and primes the lungs for breathing. There may be no more exquisite use of "stress" in nature than the positive, preparatory stress of birth.

A few years ago, commenting on the impact of monitors and the sudden redefinition of normal stress as "distress," a New York obstetrician told *Ms.* magazine, "The most common cause of Cesareans today is not fetal distress, or maternal distress, but obstetrician distress."

---

* Discussed in detail in Chapter 2.

Breech Babies: The Indians Knew the Answer

About 4 percent of all babies—and 6 percent of first babies—are breeches. Because they are more often premature and more likely to have birth defects, the mortality of breech infants is above average, but even normal-weight full-term breech babies still die too often. Cesareans have become the preferred way to deliver breeches; probably 80 to 90 percent of breeches are now delivered surgically—that's 90,000 or more babies a year—making breeches the third most frequent reason given for Cesareans.

In the case of breech babies, statistics did seem to favor changing to Cesarean in many cases. However, even though at low Cesarean rates, survival was better for normal-weight breech babies delivered by Cesarean, the Consensus Conference observed that the five-fold increase in Cesarean breech deliveries between 1970 and 1978 had not improved *overall* normal-weight breech survival. (Breech babies who weigh more than nine pounds are somewhat different and their survival is better with a Cesarean.)

No one knows why the expected improvement in total breech survival—that is, Cesarean and vaginally born babies combined—has not occurred. Perhaps, at the lower rates, doctors were already catching all breech babies for whom the delivery method—and not other problems—really spelled the difference in survival; perhaps Cesareans were just a promising, but ultimately false hope. This paradox is not only apparent in the United States. In Canada between 1973 and 1979, the Royal Victoria Hospital in Montreal changed its Cesarean delivery rate for breeches from 22 percent to 94 percent—again without reaping any improvement in the condition of normal-weight infants.

The Consensus Conference therefore concluded that vaginal delivery is still "an acceptable choice" for many normal-weight breech babies. But a more important question is whether the choice between Cesarean and vaginal delivery even addresses the problem of a breech baby. Either way, delivering an upside-down baby requires extra skill from the obstetrician, and Cesareans are not a panacea. There is, however, a way to substantially avoid breech births. An obstetrician may be able to turn the baby to its proper position weeks *before* the birth. A technique, known as external version,* takes about five minutes in experienced hands and is so simple that many people smile when they first hear about it, not quite believing that the much-debated breech dilemma could have so straightforward a solution. What happens is that the doctor places his or her hands on top of the mother's abdomen, feels for the baby's buttocks and head, and, with one hand guiding the head and the other the buttocks, carefully rotates the baby until its head is properly down.

Many ancient cultures, including American Indians, used external version for breech babies. But in the current technology of obstetrics, it has become almost a lost art. Dr. Brooks Ranney, for one, has now employed external version for more than thirty years, and his re-

* Discussed further in Chapter 3.

sults, summarized in *The American Journal of Obstetrics and Gynecology,* have helped to renew interest in this procedure. Not only did he successfully position 90 percent of the babies he tried to turn, but the enormous—tenfold—drop in their prematurity rate, and the even greater plunge in their death rate, suggests that external version may, at last, offer hopes for breech babies that Cesareans simply have not offered.

Parents whose babies are breech will want to carefully examine their choices. "I suppose the thing that surprised us most," comments one father whose breech son eventually arrived by a successful vaginal birth, "is that when we first learned that the baby hadn't turned, it was so hard to get clear information about what we should do. Whether it was doctors, books, or the instructor in our childbirth education class, we had a great deal of trouble obtaining a good idea of the risks and what factors were important for a vaginal birth, which was what we wanted. I would have thought, with breeches being so common, it would have been easier to get information; but I'm glad we went to the trouble to learn as much as we did."

Variables: Who You Are and Where You Are

In summary, it is abundantly clear that the increase in Cesarean sections in this country has scant basis in medical necessity. Unspecific medical jargon—"dystocia," "fetal distress"—should not be used to excuse the shift in our hospitals from natural births to Cesareans.

Cesareans are necessary when babies are simply too big, but American mothers are not shrinking, and in the past twenty years the average size of American infants has varied only slightly—from 7.4 to 7.6 pounds. The 98 percent Cesarean rate for repeat mothers cannot be supported by evidence. More than half—and possibly 75 percent or more—of Cesareans for fetal distress are evidently based on a wrong diagnosis. This is not to say that there aren't large babies, distressed babies, labors that just go on too long, and a multitude of other good reasons for individual Cesareans. It is not even to say that those physicians were wrong who, in the 1950s, began to advocate Cesareans not just for life-threatening emergencies, but to avoid potential emergencies such as a difficult forceps delivery; they were influenced by evidence that was valid at the time.

Parents should be aware that the nonmedical variables influencing the incidence of Cesareans fall more heavily on some women than on others. Are you a private patient? Throughout much of the United States, being a private patient makes you much more likely to have a Cesarean section than if you are a clinic patient —even though women who can afford their own physicians are generally in better health than those who can't. Or, are you from the Northeast? There are more Cesareans per capita in the Northeast than in the South, the West, or the Midwest, differences which hold true for all maternal age groups. What conceivable "medical" difference could explain why women who live in the Northeast have 30 percent more operations in childbirth than those who live in the Midwest? Perhaps the Northeast, with its concentration of medical schools, outpaces other areas, for better or worse, in shifting to new medical fads.

Unexplained variations in Cesareans do not occur

just in the United States. In Europe, countries with virtually the same infant survival rates have widely different Cesarean rates. Canada seems to have a peculiar Cesarean problem all its own. Although the Canadian government insures doctors against malpractice—and Canada does not have the many uncared-for mothers who, in the United States, form a separate high-risk obstetric population—for a time in the mid-1970s the Canadian Cesarean rate even surpassed ours, and remains the world's second highest. The average hospital stay for surgical deliveries is three days longer in Canada, and with its transfusion rate for Cesarean mothers almost 50 percent higher than in the United States, Canada might benefit from retraining its obstetricians in proper operating techniques to curtail hemorrhaging.

Costs and Challenges

The burden on medical and social resources represented by this one operation is now remarkable. At an average cost of $4,000, Cesareans consume about $2.5 billion in health dollars a year, equal to about 2 percent of the 1982 national debt. With 10 percent of Cesarean mothers requiring at least one transfusion—and, usually, two or more—they use an estimated 135,000 units of blood a year. Since all surgery in the United States requires 30,000 units a day, this is more than a four-day blood supply for the whole nation; for the greater New

York metropolitan area, it is a 130-day supply. While the individual doctor may not always realize the resources his or her own Cesarean operations require, doctors at large hospitals like Los Angeles Women's tend to just grimace or cast their eyes to heaven when they consider the strain had their Cesarean rate reached the national average; Women's Hospital would have to find operating rooms, supplies, blood, nurses, doctors, and anesthetists for seven hundred more operations a year. "I can't even think about it," one doctor comments.

But it is on parents that the challenge of the Cesarean explosion falls most heavily. They must decide what this tremendous change in obstetrics means for them and for the birth of their own baby. They must learn how to tell which doctors and hospitals are judicious in deciding when Cesareans are needed.

In New York City there is a medical complex which illustrates just how much hospitals determined to control Cesarean births can accomplish. This complex comprises two public hospitals, North Central Bronx and Bronx Municipal, and one private hospital, Einstein, whose departments of obstetrics and gynecology are affiliated with the Albert Einstein College of Medicine. In personnel and organization, the hospitals are quite different. At North Central Bronx, nurse-midwives conduct 90 percent of deliveries, probably the highest percentage of midwife births of any American hospital. Bronx Municipal is a teaching hospital where resident physicians oversee most births, and at Albert Einstein private physicians predominate. Yet all three hospitals have consistently maintained Cesarean rates below the national average and good, even outstanding infant survival. All three pioneered trial labor for previous Cesarean mothers and, as part of the emphasis on normal birth, have been highly receptive to nurse-midwives, birth assistants whose training specifically concentrates on normal deliveries.

Dr. Harold Schulman, who as chairman of the department of obstetrics and gynecology at the Albert Einstein College of Medicine from 1970 to 1979 helped supervise all three hospitals during the Cesarean explosion, summarizes their philosophy. "We could just never believe," he says, "that nature would make the mistake of constructing the female body in a way that would require surgery for one out of five women to give birth."

There is no doubt that parents who believe that surgery should not be common in childbirth can make their philosophy felt. By learning about Cesareans before the delivery, most mothers will not routinely accept a diagnosis of "dystocia" or "distress" or that they "must" have a Cesarean for second babies or breeches or other "risk" infants. "Parents today simply have to understand the reality of Cesareans," emphasizes Diony Young, a member of the board of directors of the International Childbirth Education Association. "They really must take off their rose-colored glasses and learn about this. They should never think Cesareans don't concern them."

Chapter Two

FIVE QUESTIONS THAT CUT THE PROSPECT OF SURGERY

C oncern about Cesareans is widespread, and voices from women's health groups to the National Institutes of Health have called for fewer Cesarean operations. Yet in 1981, 150,000 more Cesareans were performed in the United States than in 1980. It would seem that stabilizing Cesarean rates is a challenge as formidable as braking one of those block-long supertankers which, in its unwieldy momentum, takes some miles to stop even after the engines have been reversed. In the case of Cesareans, parents will have to be the ones to meet this challenge. "Only when women realize the awful things being perpetrated on them will Cesareans stop being abused," maintains Nancy Cohen, a widely respected birth activist and co-author of *Silent Knife*.

We are confronted with a highly abnormal situation; doctors openly admit that they do not always practice the best obstetrics because they are heavily influenced by legal considerations. Prominent physicians writing in medical journals continually protest that thousands of Cesareans performed each year are not only unnecessary, but potentially dangerous. And, for all its birth technology, its Cesareans, and its intensive-care nurseries, the United States still lags behind places like Singapore and Hong Kong in infant survival. How can parents make a difference? Parents by themselves cannot expect to entirely change American birth practices, but they can crucially influence the way their own babies are born, and especially, they can take major steps to avoid unnecessary Cesareans.

An important first step is to ask the five basic questions which should be central to the parents' choice of where, how, and by whom—an obstetrician, family practitioner, midwife—their baby is delivered. Unfortunately, most people spend more time shopping for a new suit or dress than for a doctor and hospital for childbirth. Asking questions will require some work and research; but parents will find few more rewarding experiences in life than spending the time to be sure a birth is both happy and safe.

The five basic questions that follow are designed for mothers who anticipate normal pregnancies* and deliveries; used intelligently, these questions can easily halve the general prospect of having an unnecessary Cesarean. Remember, the majority of women who end up with Cesareans did, in fact, have what appeared to be very normal pregnancies all along, so it is crucial for all mothers to think carefully about a hospital's Cesarean policies. Perhaps the most common protest after a Cesarean is, "But I don't understand it. I'm in such good health and nothing like this has ever happened to me."

---

* Detailed considerations for mothers with known "problem pregnancies"—diabetics, those with herpes, a previous Cesarean, twins, etc.—are discussed in Chapter 3.

In case an unexpected problem does develop toward the end of the pregnancy—a breech or overdue infant perhaps—these questions will have also proved invaluable by having directed the parents to professionals who do not automatically resort to Cesarean to solve problems. When problems occur, it is more important than ever to have thoroughly investigated the options and have confidence that the doctor will treat you and your baby as individuals—not as part of a medical fad.

Cesarean rates are not, of course, the sole factor to consider in choosing a birth attendant and hospital; parents will also want to review a hospital's safety record, its general atmosphere and facilities, and to feel very comfortable with the doctor or midwife. Yet no other issue in contemporary obstetrics can more quickly reveal whether a hospital will be candid about its own practices and whether a doctor has kept up to date with medical research and is willing to discuss controversial issues.

1. What Are the Cesarean Rates of the Hospital and the Physician?

Cesarean rates can fluctuate tremendously from hospital to hospital within the same community. In 1980, for example, Cesarean rates within New York City ranged from 9.2 percent of births at North Central Bronx Hospital to 24 percent at prestigious New York Hospital to 36.7 percent at Brooklyn's Interboro Hospital. Even on Staten Island, where most mothers are healthy middle-class women, Cesarean rates varied, from 17.9 percent of births at Staten Island Hospital to 32.4 percent at Richmond Memorial Hospital—a startling figure for a hospital which does not serve a high-risk population. Obviously, an informed mother on Staten Island could almost halve her prospects for a Cesarean by choosing between the two hospitals.

Similarly, in 1977 on Long Island, Cesareans ranged from 7.7 percent of births at Central Suffolk Hospital to 25.7 percent at Southampton Hospital—even though the patients at Southampton, who live in a radiant resort and farming area, presumably enjoy good health, certainly more so than those at Central Suffolk Hospital, who are much less affluent. And these unusual fluctuations are not peculiar to the Eastern states. In Washington State, published rates for 1977 show Cesareans at 10.4 percent of births at Madigan Army Hospital, 12.5 percent at the Group Health Cooperative of Puget Sound, and 16.8 percent at Kaiser-Portland Hospital. Such variations occur in communities across the country, and among hospitals serving mothers who do not differ in terms of risk or general health. It is a mindless phenomenon, and one to be on guard for when investigating hospitals.

To obtain a hospital's Cesarean rate, ask at the obstetrics department or the public relations or patient representative office at the hospital. Cesarean rates are also often available from state or local health departments, but if a hospital is unwilling to reveal such basic information, this may be a sign that you will never receive the cooperation you have every right to expect during your baby's birth.

Outside urban areas, your choice of hospitals will be somewhat limited, but even then you may have more options than you think. Check with friends, the state hospital directory, nurse-midwife associations, and any other appropriate health organizations listed in your telephone directory and investigate *every* facility within a reasonable distance—perhaps up to one hour's traveling—from your home. Some parents willingly travel even farther if they are dissatisfied with local facilities.

Checking Hospital Safety

Of course, parents will want to know more about a hospital than just its Cesarean rates. Other important issues are whether the hospital allows fathers and other family members or friends to be present in the delivery room, whether it encourages mothers to handle their babies right away, and whether there is rooming-in, so that the baby can be with the mother and not in a nursery. Most important, parents will want to assure themselves of the hospital's safety and competence— reassurance which can be obtained in part by studying infant mortality rates.

Infant mortality is usually divided into three categories: perinatal deaths, those which occur between the fifth month of pregnancy and the first month after birth; neonatal deaths, those within one month after the delivery; and infant deaths, those within a year of birth. Perinatal deaths and neonatal deaths are most closely related to the care the mother received before and during delivery; neonatal deaths alone give a sufficient indication of how well babies fare within a short time of delivery.

In comparing survival rates, however, it is crucial to be aware that, as much as hospital and physician care, the health of the mothers affects infant survival and can vary a great deal. While one hospital would be expected to have good infant survival simply because the mothers who use it are robustly healthy, another hospital a few miles away which serves high-risk mothers might still be doing well even though its survival statistics are not as impressive. Two factors in particular to consider are whether a hospital serves large numbers of minority mothers and of mothers who have not had prenatal care. Since neonatal deaths are about twice the average rate for both these groups, the hospital's survival rates would suffer—again, even though it may be doing well in terms of its patient population.

Some hospitals that give out their Cesarean rate will nonetheless balk at telling parents their infant mortality rate. They may claim that parents "can't understand" the factors involved. It may then be easier to simply obtain these various statistics—neonatal mortality, the percentage of mothers lacking prenatal care, and so forth—from your state or local health department. (It is not, by the way, very useful to try to compare infant mortality rates between individual doctors. Doctors don't handle enough deliveries every year to provide valid statistics, and the bad luck of having had just a few patients who, through no one's fault, lost their babies could distort an entire year's record.)

Again, these are rough comparisons, but perhaps the most important thing parents will learn from looking at infant survival and Cesarean rates together is how often hospitals with low Cesarean rates do actually boast good infant survival. We have already discussed a few outstanding hospitals—Los Angeles Women's, Denver General, North Central Bronx—where this is the case. For more reassurance, let's look at a few studies which have compared hospitals in large geographic areas. The 1977 study of Long Island hospitals, for example, pinpointed three large hospitals—Mercy, Nassau Mineola, and St. Charles Good Samaritan—each of which numbered more than 1,500 annual deliveries and between 10 and 11 percent minority mothers. St. Charles Good Samaritan, with the lowest Cesarean rate (14.2 percent), had the best neonatal mortality rate (5.5 per 1,000 live births), while Nassau Mineola, with the highest Cesarean rate, 23.2 percent, had a neonatal mortality rate of 6.2 per 1,000. Mercy Hospital, with a 16 percent Cesarean rate, had a neonatal mortality rate of 7.6 per 1,000. In New York City in 1980, the six public hospitals with the lowest Cesarean rates had lower average neonatal and perinatal mortality than the six public hospitals with the highest Cesarean rates. And among private hospitals in Manhattan, the three with the lowest Cesarean rates all achieved above-average infant survival for private hospitals, even while serving a full share of minority mothers and mothers lacking prenatal care.

In short, by looking for hospitals with low Cesarean rates, parents will often be rewarded by finding hospitals which also have excellent safety records. This does not mean that there are not some "bad" hospitals with low Cesarean rates; there are. But on the whole, hospitals appear to achieve low Cesarean rates because they are well-run places. Their success does not come by chance, but because they know how to deliver babies well.

Choosing the Right Doctor

The record of the doctor who will perform the delivery is also crucial. To some extent, hospital policies can influence an individual doctor's Cesarean rate. If the hospital won't permit the doctor to try normal deliveries for previous Cesarean mothers or breech deliveries, or if it doesn't have the laboratory facilities for fetal scalp sampling, the doctor is stuck. Nonetheless, the individual Cesarean rates of doctors working at the same hospital—and delivering mothers who are identical in health—can fluctuate so widely it almost takes the breath away. In *The American Journal of Obstetrics and Gynecology,* Dr. Robert Sack discussed a suburban Los Angeles hospital with five staff obstetricians; their individual Cesarean rates ranged from 16 percent to 40 percent of the births under their care!

Clearly, parents should know a doctor's Cesarean rate and his or her attitude about the whole Cesarean question. To get this information, you will have to ask. Ask politely and considerately, but by all means *ask,* because it is unlikely that the doctor will initiate such a conversation.

"The hope, usually unfulfilled, may be that the obstetrician will at some time during the pregnancy draw up a chair and talk about his or her perceptions of birth and how it will be handled, the hospital set-up and respective roles of parent and obstetrician," Constance A. Bean, a health educator at the Massachusetts Institute of Technology, writes in *Methods of Childbirth.* "However, the couple will in almost every case be required to take the initiative. Questions eliciting attitude are useful. 'How do you feel about routine episiotomies [incisions to "widen" the vagina]?' 'What do you think of [alternative] birthing rooms?' 'How do you feel about the increased Cesarean rate?' "

Aside from the doctor's Cesarean rate, it is just as important to inquire about his or her attitude toward routine interventions which sometimes lead to unnecessary Cesareans. Electronic monitoring and automatic intravenouses, by forcing the mother to keep still and preventing her from walking, work against the natural progress of labor; even as minor a routine procedure as an enema may hardly be helpful. "We never give routine enemas," explains a midwife at North Central Bronx, "because we want mothers to feel in control of themselves and their labor right from the beginning, while enemas make people feel out of control." Episiotomies, although performed toward the end of labor, may also loom as a prospect that makes some mothers feel tense or frightened.

If the doctor is reluctant to discuss his own Cesarean rate and policies on electronic monitors, episiotomies, and other procedures, or if he seems unwilling to consider your views, it is a pretty good sign that the whole relationship will never be comfortable or candid. "I do think," states Kris Berger, a Wichita, Kansas, mother who counsels parents for the Peace and Home Association of Wichita, a natural-childbirth advocacy group, "that people give up a little too easily. For instance, I recently had a couple who came from outside Wichita. Two doctors had told them 'no way' could the mother, who'd had a Cesarean, expect a vaginal delivery; but we found three doctors willing to help them try."

When interviewing an obstetrician—and that's what you are doing, because you will be employing him—it helps to be well prepared. Read and study about birth and have a list of questions ready. For instance, after Kris Berger's first child, a breech, was born by Cesarean, she studied her options for vaginal delivery for over a year before she even thought of getting pregnant with her second baby. She read books and sent away to several Cesarean support groups for literature, and finally made up a three-page typed list of questions to ask the doctors she interviewed. "Actually," she laughs, "that did turn out to be a little much, so I boiled it down to essentials and would ask the main points on the phone before deciding to see them personally. Reactions ranged from understanding to the implication that I needed psychotherapy. One doctor who was the nicest on the phone was the worst in person. All told, I interviewed seven doctors personally and, in the end, I didn't even really have to interview the one I chose. He just outrightly told me what his philosophy of birth was—which fit with mine. He tries to make a hospital birth as close to a home birth as possible, with no routine interventions, and the mother helping to pull the baby out and the father cutting the cord. He's very easy to talk to. I bring him articles and he reads them and makes comments."

If possible, mothers should conduct this search with their husband, a friend, or a relative. It is always helpful to have another person's thoughts about such a major decision, but most important, the willingness of health professionals to answer questions usually increases in proportion to the number of people in the room. You can start by asking friends to recommend an obstetrician, but you should also consider contacting local childbirth education and activist groups. These may include the La Leche League, widely known for its encouragement of breast-feeding, and the recently formed Cesarean Prevention Movement, which has chapters in several states and is growing rapidly. Usually, these groups can supply lists of local doctors who emphasize natural birth.

Remember that not only obstetricians deliver babies. The choices also include a midwife, a family practitioner, or a general practitioner. Possibly the most ill-advised choice is a gynecologist who only delivers babies as an occasional sideline. A survey conducted by the American College of Obstetrics and Gynecology found that when at least 75 percent of their caseload was concentrated on obstetrics, the doctors replying had an average Cesarean rate of 24 percent; when most of their time was spent on gynecology, doctors who also delivered babies had a whopping 54 percent Cesarean rate!

Finally, trust your instincts. Mothers should, above all, feel comfortable and confident about a doctor. This is the time to listen to the voice in the back of your head that says "I wonder about this." Don't think you can eventually talk a doctor into your way of thinking.

In the first place, pregnancy is not a time for prolonged arguments. In the second place, there is no reason why all doctors should practice obstetrics precisely alike. Attitudes and policies that you don't like may be what the next mother wants, so just calmly take yourself elsewhere.

Private or Group Practice?

Parents who wish to have their baby delivered by a private physician, and who have in mind the heroic Norman Rockwell image of the lone obstetrician struggling, tired but determined, long through the night to deliver yet another inconveniently timed baby, will be well advised to think again. While there are, unquestionably, outstanding physicians who manage the exhausting and unrelenting demands of a private obstetric practice, considerable opinion views this traditional practice of obstetrics as self-defeating. Dr. Harold Schulman, now chief of obstetrics at Bronx Municipal Hospital, and who also practices privately with a group of obstetricians and midwives, finds the physician working alone the least effective method of organizing an obstetrical practice. "Consider," Dr. Schulman points out, "that this doctor has an office separate from the hospital and he's probably affiliated with at least two hospitals anyway. So there he is running between three places. He's tired and makes a bad decision because of that. In addition, the pressure of having to be someplace else for another delivery may lead him to cut some births short and do a Cesarean too soon."

Group practice offers parents a way to have a private physician and yet be protected from the distractions and the sheer exhaustion associated with the individual practice of obstetrics. Usually, group practices are arranged so that a mother sees the same doctor for her prenatal care. However, the doctors take turns standing by for night deliveries. "This arrangement really cuts the fatigue element," Dr. Schulman emphasizes, "by letting the obstetrician count on some regular nights when he can get some sleep and someone he knows is assigned to cover for him."

As your delivery date approaches, you can prepare by introducing yourself to other doctors in the group, particularly those scheduled for night duty. It is also crucial, at this time, to be sure that any special plans you have discussed with your own doctor—your preferences regarding routine drugs and electronic monitoring, rooming-in with the baby, and having your own childbirth coach or "labor support" person at the delivery—are in writing and will be given to the delivery doctor when you begin labor. As an added precaution, have your doctor make a copy of these special instructions for you to bring to the hospital. Too often, comments one birth educator, "the doctor has said, 'Yeah, yeah, everyone understands what you want,' and it turns out, at the hospital, that nobody does."

Some parents may veer away from group practice because they want to be sure their own doctor, and not a "stranger," delivers their baby. Yet, it may be to your advantage to have a different doctor for the delivery. "When a doctor knows the family well, the more he may want to show them he is doing something for them

when there's a difficulty," comments the chief of obstetrics of a large Eastern hospital. "You can just see it
happening. There's the father pacing around and the
mother wondering what's going on and there's the doctor thinking, 'I'm going to have to face these people for
the rest of my life if something goes wrong.' It's only
human, but I don't think it increases objectivity about
when to perform a Cesarean."

Once again, each mother has to decide what is important to her—a personal physician or, potentially, a
less harried, more objective delivery. In any case, do
remember that at public hospitals such as Los Angeles
Women's, Denver General and North Central Bronx,
which are doing so well with both infant survival and
Cesarean rates, no mother has her "own" doctor.

2. Does the Hospital Require Peer Review or Second Opinions for Cesareans?

Once every month at St. Vincent's Hospital, which
had the lowest Cesarean rate in 1980 of any Manhattan
private hospital, doctors from the obstetrics department gather for a conference on Cesarean section. Residents and experienced staff doctors receive a summary
of the month's obstetric surgery. For an hour and a half,
cases are discussed and the doctors must justify for
their peers why each operation was performed. "We

started the special monthly conference in 1977 when we saw Cesarean rates zooming all around us and we wanted to be sure that we ourselves weren't performing unnecessary surgery," explains Dr. Jerome Dolan, who recently retired as St. Vincent's chief of obstetrics. "I consider it absolutely crucial in having helped us to control our Cesarean rate."

The conviction that peer review may be the most important step toward controlling Cesareans is widely shared. At public hospitals, which are usually teaching institutions, shared decisions and consultation for Cesareans are automatic; a Cesarean decision would typically involve a first-, second-, and third-year resident, the chief resident, and, finally, require the permission of the chief or director of obstetrics. In addition, large public hospitals usually have full-time perinatologists, specialists in the condition of babies during the birth period, who would also be consulted before deciding on a Cesarean. In interviews, all directors of obstetrics of New York City's public hospitals cited the process of shared decision-making as the major factor in curbing their Cesarean rates—in fact, more important even than the relative freedom from malpractice pressures in public medicine.

At most private hospitals, doctors can perform Cesareans on their patients without consultation or second opinions; consultation is usual only when the hospital is also training residents and has assigned them clinic patients. Or, there may be token consultations of no real practical value. "Peer review should mean real review, not window dressing," emphasizes Dr. Schulman. "These opinions have to be given carefully and in person. Einstein has been one of the few private hospitals I know of where the rules for consultation for clinic and private patients are the same. We don't have guys calling another doctor on the phone and saying, 'Well, here's the story. Give me a green light.' And we don't have guys running in at the last minute and saying, 'Oh, let's do a Cesarean.' "

Consultation Improves Infant Health

Aside from its value in controlling the Cesarean rate, consultation is equally important in improving obstetrics. It seems obvious that when a delivery becomes problematic, the combined expertise of two or more specialists is more likely to assure the correct decision for both mother and baby. Here is where a second opinion might help find the safest course for an overdue baby; or another doctor might caution against scheduling an early Cesarean, to allow more time for the fetal lungs to mature in the womb.

These are no small matters to the health of babies. The Neonatal Intensive Care Unit at Hershey Medical Center, a regional care center which takes in the sickest newborns from forty-two "feeder" hospitals in central Pennsylvania, has reported that over a period of three years, *every single baby transferred there with severe respiratory distress following a prematurely performed Cesarean was delivered by a private physician.* In no case had the attending obstetrician, acting alone, made a special effort, including consultation, to determine the correct gestational age of the infant. Almost certainly, consultation prior to Cesareans was a factor in preventing any *clinic* baby from the forty-two hospitals from developing severe respiratory distress attributable to a badly timed Cesarean.

If your hospital doesn't require consultation for Cesareans, you can arrange with your doctor beforehand to request a second opinion if during the delivery it appears that a Cesarean might be necessary; only in a rare emergency would there not be enough time. But you may find that in hospitals where consultation is not already accepted, the response will be hostile at best and that any consultation is done grudgingly and hastily. Hospitals which do not recognize the value of peer review may not want to bother with the follow-through necessary in enforcing standards for the private physicians who use their facility. Also, at many hospitals, especially small, private hospitals, the doctors are part-owners of the facility and able to stop the administration from pressing the issue.

3. Does the Hospital Use Fetal Scalp-Blood Sampling?

There is simply no doubt that scalp-blood sampling can dramatically reduce the number of Cesareans performed needlessly when doctors misinterpret fetal monitors. Depending on the stage of labor in which "suspicious" heartbeat variations appear on the monitor, between 50 and 90 percent of infants will still have normal blood chemistry, a more accurate indication of their condition. "What obstetrics hasn't learned very well," Dr. Schulman says of the current situation, "is to distinguish between the normal stress of birth and 'distress.' "

Yet scalp-blood sampling is not widely used. As we have seen, in New York City, even with its concentration of medical schools, only seventeen of the fifty-five hospitals with obstetrics services used scalp sampling for at least 1 percent of births in 1980. While it is difficult to suggest an "ideal" scalp sampling rate, it is also hard to see, with 5 percent of Cesareans being performed for presumed "distress," that a 1 percent rate begins to tap its advantages.

Why isn't scalp sampling employed more often? The standard excuse is that hospitals don't have the laboratory facilities. However, laboratory facilities are, after all, part of what hospitals are supposed to supply. "Sometimes it is the labs. But the basic problem has been that doctors don't want to do it. They weren't trained when they were residents and they don't bother to learn now," comments Dr. Edward Quilligan, the former chief of obstetrics who marshaled Los Angeles Women's Hospital through the Cesarean explosion.

Why so many doctors will undertake a major operation but not attempt a two-minute test is a question best left to a philosophy course on the values of Western medicine. In the meantime, parents are well advised to learn about the scalp sampling capability of the hospital they choose.

4. Does the Hospital Employ Nurse-Midwives and Alternative Birth Rooms?

Many hospitals with low Cesarean rates use nurse-midwives to supervise their normal or "low risk" deliveries. Hospitals which welcome midwives now often set them up in an "alternative birth room" which is inside the hospital, but where parents are free from the intrusive and intimidating routines typical of medical birth. New mothers are delighted that their babies were delivered by someone who believed childbirth should be a natural, joyful, and memorable experience. "The midwife just talked me through it," explained one previous Cesarean mother after giving birth normally to her second child.

In contrast to the training of physicians, which focuses heavily on the pathology and emergencies of pregnancy, the training of nurse-midwives emphasizes the normalcy of childbirth. Midwives try to avoid the uncomfortable and sometimes painful procedures which most doctors perform automatically during labor. Midwives, for example, don't give enemas, intravenouses, or episiotomies unless there is a medical need. They try to support the mother in her own natural rhythms of birth—they believe the mother, and not medical personnel, should be in control. They look to natural ways, including close emotional support and "verbal anesthesia," to encourage a good labor. "We don't call women in labor 'patients,'" explains one Texas midwife. "We just call them 'the mothers' or 'the ladies.' When you call someone a patient it sounds as though they're ill and, of course, giving birth is not an illness."

But even more important, the *safety* of hospital-based midwife services is unparalleled. North Central Bronx, Kings County Hospital in Brooklyn, the Frontier Nursing Service of Leslie County, Kentucky, and Los Angeles Women's Hospital all have high percentages of midwife deliveries, and all serve high-risk mothers. Yet all are nationally known for their good infant survival. They also boast strikingly low Cesarean rates; only 2 percent of the 3,000 annual births supervised by midwives at the Normal Birth Center of Women's Hospital are Cesareans.

The use of midwives increases birth safety in another important way. When midwives handle a hospital's normal births, they free doctors to concentrate on problem pregnancies and occasional emergencies. At North Central Bronx, staffed by fifteen nurse-midwives and twelve obstetricians, the midwives handle all normal deliveries—about 90 percent. Interestingly, when the hospital opened in 1977, the midwives, like many doctors, at first thought the ideal arrangement would be to assign each mother an individual midwife for both her prenatal care and delivery. This approach fell by the wayside a month after the service started—for much the same reasons that the individual practice of obstetrics is so difficult. "With two thousand deliveries a year," comments Theresa Dondero, the head midwife, "it was too hard to organize. Everyone was getting tired and distracted from being called in at unscheduled hours for deliveries, which then interfered with their scheduled prenatal appointments. So we decided to assign mothers to a group."

With a rotating staff, midwives and obstetricians are on the premises at North Central Bronx around the clock. In emergencies this team is already on hand and there are no scenes of confusion and panic as the mother's doctor is summoned from bed or dinner and then forced into hasty decisions the minute he reaches the hospital. The rewards for this approach have been huge. North Central Bronx, aside from its low Cesarean rate, has for years maintained the best infant survival of any public hospital in New York—and survival there also outranks the average for clinic deliveries at the city's private hospitals. "What's interesting," notes Theresa Dondero, "is that we never set out with the goal of a low Cesarean rate. We were a little surprised ourselves when the figures started coming in; it came about because we were doing other things right."

However, many hospitals still intensely oppose hiring midwives. This opposition is disheartening. The United States is one of the few countries where hospitals routinely bar midwives. But there are many midwives, as there are obstetricians, who think it almost impossible to conduct a relaxed, natural birth in the noise and tension of a hospital environment. As a result, in recent years in the United States "birthing centers" have become an exciting new alternative for parents and medical personnel alike who believe in normal birth.

A Growing Alternative: The Birthing Center

Birthing centers are small, homelike facilities where mothers deliver in a normal bed, instead of being strapped to the cold steel of a delivery table. They may eat as they wish, have visits from family and friends, and labor in any position that seems comfortable. Usually the mother, alert from a normal, nonanesthetized labor, leaves for home with her baby within a few hours of the birth. Mothers receive all their prenatal care at the center, and a full-care package, including classes in prepared childbirth and consultation with both an obstetrician and pediatrician, costs about one-half as much as a hospital birth.

About 150 birthing centers, half of them run by midwives with doctors as consultants and the other half started by doctors, are now functioning in the United States. While many have not been open long enough to establish a safety record (and the American College of Obstetricians and Gynecologists opposes any form of "out-of-hospital" births), there is no reason to think that the general safety of birthing centers isn't perfectly reassuring. In the first place, these centers carefully screen out mothers with potential problems, and they also have backup arrangements with local hospitals. In the second place, the record of the oldest centers is enviable. The birthing center at Manhattan's Maternity Center Association, the oldest in the country, has not encountered a single life-threatening emergency since opening in 1975; mortality for babies born at the Clinica Familiar (Family Clinic) of Raymondville, Texas, is below the average for Texas hospitals. The midwives there have established this excellent record even though, because they serve a mostly rural and poor population an hour's drive from the nearest hospital, they cannot be as strict as most in sending high-risk mothers to doctors from the start.

A survey of the longer established centers, recently published in the journal *Lancet*, suggested that the Cesarean rate for mothers accepted at centers is about 5 percent; the women were, of course, transferred to a hospital for the operation itself.

"I'll tell you who really benefited, in my opinion," comments Anne Strickland Squadron, a New York mother who had her second baby at the Maternity Center Association's center. "I think the baby benefited. The birth was so gentle. He got an easy, nice start. The first time, I had about as nonobtrusive a hospital birth as you can get—I didn't have any medication, monitoring, or an IV—but still, the hospital routine kept intruding. They separated me from the baby for two hours to stay in the recovery room, and they kept me in the hospital for three days, which was totally unnecessary. Let me give an example. My labor really slowed when I got to the center. The midwife suggested an enema. I asked what that would do and she said it would speed the birth, so I agreed; and it worked, too. But there was nothing automatic or threatening about it. I think in the hospital, when labor slows, so often the control of the birth is taken away from the mother. Next thing, she's given Pitocin, then she's put on a monitor, then she's headed toward a Cesarean. The way this was handled at the birthing center struck me as being a medically sound, conservative way."

Once again, however, each mother has to determine where her own greatest comfort and confidence lie; some women want hospitals, just as others find hospitals threatening and nerve-wracking. "If you have a birthing center near you, just visit and check it out," Anne Squadron advises. "Once you see how it operates, you may decide it is more right for you than you imagined."

5. Does a Hospital Have Rigid Rules for Cesarean Decisions?

Many hospitals have an inflexible set of rules (referred to as protocols), either stated or implied, which obstetricians are expected to follow in making a decision to do a Cesarean section. While all hospitals need guidelines for safety, rigid protocols do not take into consideration the condition of the individual mother and infant.

In some hospitals all mothers are given an intravenous drip of glucose water, even when there is no medical reason; not only is the drip uncomfortable, but once she is attached to the intravenous needle, the hospital may then forbid the mother to walk at all and demand she use a bedpan. If she is not comfortable about this, and fails to urinate frequently, her labor may slow and an unnecessary Cesarean may then be ordered. Or the doctor may routinely break the membranes of the amniotic sac surrounding the baby early in labor; then, because the hospital fears infection after the baby loses this protective shield, it will demand delivery within a certain number of hours, sometimes as few as eight or twelve. As a result, the mother may end up with a Cesarean which never would have occurred if the sac had been left to rupture by itself or not been ruptured until she was well dilated. Similarly, hospitals may use Pitocin, the synthetic hormone, to stimulate labor almost routinely. While Pitocin sometimes helps in labors that are halting or weak, its unnecessary use can cause overstrong contractions which send the baby into distress, again necessitating a Cesarean which wouldn't have been needed otherwise.

Although the average first labor is twelve to fourteen hours long, and plenty go on longer, some obstetric departments perform Cesareans on virtually all mothers whose labor lasts beyond twelve hours. (A generation ago, labor lasting twenty-four to thirty-six hours, or longer, was not even considered worth remarking. Just for reassurance, ask your mother how long her first labor was.) Some hospitals won't perform any vaginal breech deliveries at all; others induce labor—with Cesareans often following—for virtually all postmature pregnancies, usually defined as those which last longer than forty-two weeks.

"I know I wouldn't want to be treated by a protocol," Dr. Ranney comments, "so why should anyone else? Care should be individual and for that mother. The only reason for protocol medicine is to keep partially trained individuals from making mistakes, so I don't admire it. Gradually, people's judgment atrophies and they stop thinking."

Arbitrary Time Limits; Arbitrary Monitoring

Protocols about monitoring and length of labor probably result in the most Cesareans. Often, decisions about length of labor are based on Friedman's Curve, a pattern of labor stages and timing proposed by Dr. Emanuel Friedman, an obstetrician at Beth Israel Hospital in Boston and professor at the Harvard Medical School who has made it his life's work to study literally thousands of labors. Because of the association of Friedman's Curve with Cesarean section, the term is often said with a kind of hiss by believers in natural childbirth; oddly, however, Friedman's original work, which severely castigated doctors for too often causing fetal injury and death by premature attempts to remove the baby with forceps (today Cesareans, rather than forceps, would be the "removal" method), is among the most scathing in the medical literature in its view toward medical interference in labor. Indeed, it would almost seem that Dr. Friedman has obtained his large following in obstetrics because no one has ever read him; all they know are textbook summaries of his labor graphs.

Perhaps most important for mothers to realize is that Friedman did not even describe the latent phase of the first stage of labor as "abnormally prolonged" until twenty hours had passed; this latent phase, which is the time between the first clear contractions and the start of dilation of the cervix, accounts for most diagnoses of "prolonged" labor. However, even when labor was, by his own definition, abnormally prolonged, only for an arrest of labor with well-documented disproportion did Friedman advocate an immediate Cesarean, rather than first trying the natural strategies of rest, liquids, and "much needed emotional encouragement" to restart the labor. Friedman also repeatedly pointed out that a large portion of prolonged labor is caused by oversedation and anesthesia—in other words, by doctors themselves—and that the best course in such cases usually is to let the mother rest until the medication wears off and stops blocking labor progress.

Parents, in short, might often be on better ground quoting Friedman's work to argue against a Cesarean than doctors would be to argue for one. Still, on a practical level, many parents might find it easier to question rules about monitoring than to argue the technicalities of labor curves. Here, if the pregnancy has been normal, parents may find their own doctor does not agree with constant electronic monitoring—and certainly not with the obtrusive internal monitoring which requires that an electrode be attached to the baby's scalp. But the time for this discussion is before the delivery; on reaching the hospital, parents should already be armed with written instructions from their own physician for modified or no monitoring.

Research at Denver General, at the Davis Medical Center birthing room, and many other places strongly suggests that monitoring blocks good, relaxed labor. Even if that were not the case, monitoring obviously interferes with walking, an activity well documented to improve the quality of labor. At the Birmingham Maternity Hospital in Birmingham, England, women who were allowed to walk for just two and a half hours during the first stage of labor not only labored for two and a half hours less than women kept lying in bed, but none of these thirty-four women needed a Cesarean or forceps delivery and twenty completed the delivery without any drugs. All of the thirty-four women kept in bed used drugs, and eleven had forceps or Cesarean deliveries. The babies in the walking group also had better Apgar scores—all told, benefits surpassing anything monitoring has to offer most pregnancies.

Antenatal Diagnosis, a 1979 National Institutes of Health report, concluded that because monitoring is controversial and unproved, doctors should not intimidate women into agreeing to it. Nonetheless, even the most normal, low-risk mothers may find that doctors or hospital staff go almost berserk when they refuse monitoring. If opposition is total, perhaps the mother is better off seeking a compromise; North Central Bronx, for instance, with its high-risk population, monitors most—although by no means all—mothers for twenty minutes when they first arrive. Those with normal patterns are then freed from the machines.

How Mothers Can Try to "Normalize" Their Own Deliveries

Leaving aside physical exigencies, such as true disproportion or a prolapsed umbilical cord, women can significantly contribute to keeping their labor on a normal course. After you have asked your questions about the hospital and the doctor or birth attendant, and as the pregnancy progresses, you will want to learn about your own role in birth.

Childbirth Education

One of the best ways of learning to control labor is through childbirth education—or "prepared childbirth"—emphasizing relaxation and breathing techniques. At Evanston Hospital in Evanston, Illinois, five hundred women trained in the Lamaze method of childbirth were compared with five hundred women, closely matched in age, education level, and other characteristics, who did not receive any special preparation for giving birth. The trained mothers ended up having only one-fourth the number of Cesarean sections (sixteen versus sixty) and their babies had one-fifth the incidence of fetal distress. Lamaze mothers, possibly because preparation helped them to relax, also rarely went into premature labor, a factor in the significantly better perinatal survival of their babies.

As dramatic and exciting as such results are, however, they also need qualification. Diony Young, among other people, points out that although childbirth education may help avoid Cesareans, its potential in this respect is often blunted by the unwillingness of childbirth educators to confront the Cesarean explosion. "The instructors," she says, "are usually nurses, who may not be comfortable challenging a doctor or a hospital. They gloss over what has happened in obstetrics.

Some seem to have trouble even saying the word 'Cesarean.' They call it 'abdominal delivery' or 'just another way of having a baby.' At a minimum, parents should be taught about the major indications for Cesareans, instructed to ask the doctor the precise indication for a Cesarean recommended to them, and told to ask for a second opinion."

On the other hand, some childbirth education classes can cause their own set of problems. With the intention of not scaring mothers, they sometimes make natural labor seem too easy. If severe pain starts, women not prepared for it panic. "If I had one bit of advice to give," comments Carol Hagin, the Walnut Creek, California, midwife, "it's to take the attitude that childbirth is just part of being a woman. Mothers should not try to make birth into a monument, and childbirth classes sometimes glorify birth out of proportion. I've had seven children myself, and I can tell you that it's not all glorious. It was painful sometimes and there were times in labor when I just wanted to give up. Then what you need is not slogans, but someone to sit there and encourage you—what I call verbal anesthesia."

There are now several widely taught methods of prepared childbirth, including the Lamaze, Dick-Read, and Bradley methods, which differ somewhat in emphasis and approach. It's up to women to decide which method best satisfies their own vision of childbirth. Once again, however, you have to be sure that the obstetrician or attendant you choose also believes in prepared childbirth. The medical journals are full of complaints from doctors about the number of women who "fail" at natural childbirth, causing more trouble for doctors as they bitterly concede to drugs, episiotomies, and other procedures. The tone of these articles implies that somehow the doctor has nothing to do with the failures—it is all the fault of a dreamy childbirth education movement and women who are unrealistic about birth. Yet when a birth attendant fully believes in natural labor, even women without training readily achieve a normal, drug-free birth.

At North Central Bronx, 20 percent of women take childbirth education classes. While this figure disproved predictions that it was useless to expect people from rough parts of the Bronx to travel at night for a class about babies, it does leave the midwives to guide the rest of the mothers through labor with only encouragement and hastily taught breathing techniques. In an obstetrics department which believes in normal birth, the mothers summon astounding determination, and 80 percent of them—almost certainly a record for an American hospital—have drug-free deliveries. Further, the whole experience is so satisfying to them over "standard" delivery procedures that the hospital enjoys an outstanding reputation and, in an area of the city where people really don't expect much from hospitals, it attracts hundreds more mothers than it can take.

Medication and Anesthesia: More Crucial Than They Tell You

The arguments for drug-free deliveries are straightforward. In the first place, it is simply better for the

baby not to be exposed to drugs. Second, not only do
all major forms of anesthesia now used in childbirth
"slow labor and increase the number of operative deliveries" (as summarized in a recent discussion in *The
American Journal of Obstetrics and Gynecology*), but
even innocuous medications such as aspirin can unexpectedly interfere with the progress of labor. Yet it is
also pointless for the few women who do have severe
and debilitating pain to suffer through childbirth without any relief.

Learning to make intelligent decisions about medication and anesthesia is another important step a
mother can take toward controlling her labor. There is
no need for a woman to feel ashamed of reaching her
limit; what is important is that she is not pressured into
taking medication or anesthesia that she really doesn't
want. Since dispensing pain relief is one of the most
common functions of hospital personnel, they may feel
almost compelled to draw you into their routine. One
mother who delivered at a large teaching hospital remembers the anesthesia residents "practically breathing down my neck" throughout the delivery as they
kept asking if she really didn't want an epidural now.
Discuss this crucial issue with your doctor ahead of
time so there won't be any last-minute surprises for
either of you.

If you take medication to relieve pain during labor,
it should be dispensed very judiciously. Even aspirin
sometimes does more harm than good. In the early
1970s, Australian researchers startled the world of obstetrics by reporting that women who used aspirin frequently tended to have overdue babies, with the

attendant increase in Cesareans and other problems. American research has also documented average labors of five hours longer in women who use aspirin *daily* than in women who don't. Aspirin, medical science now realizes, interferes with the prostaglandins, substances which help regulate the length of gestation and labor. If these observations do not forbid all aspirin use during pregnancy—for women with arthritis or other painful diseases, aspirin still may be preferable to other drugs—they are a sharp reminder of the serious gaps in research into drug effects on the course of labor.

The "special" problems of older mothers during labor may also partly derive from drug effects. In a fascinating example of the research into true labor dysfunction—which should have preceded the Cesarean revolution, not followed it—Dr. Robert Sokol and a group at the University of Rochester School of Medicine observed that half the women over age forty-five they studied who had abnormally prolonged labor had gone into the abnormal pattern *right after* they were given the narcotic meperidine, commonly known as Demerol; no mothers under age thirty experienced abnormal labor after taking meperidine. The Sokol group concluded that "active labor is more sensitive to this drug in the elderly [mother]." But the trouble may also be that the doctors were too "sensitive" to older mothers; they consistently prescribed higher narcotic doses for mothers over age forty-five—an average dose of 73 versus 58 milligrams. You can easily see how important it is to have discussed the whole issue of medication with your doctor before you arrive at the hospital.

Yet, conversely, for the few mothers with extremely painful labor, adequate pain relief may provide the support which helps assure a normal delivery. In *Methods of Childbirth,* Constance Bean deftly summarizes a process of easing into pain relief. "Medications, in the more conservative manner, do have a place in childbirth," she writes. "They are used most effectively when an informed couple makes the decision. A small dose of Demerol (about 25 milligrams) or perhaps a tranquilizer is the usual preference. A common time to assess the possible need for drugs is at approximately 5 centimeters of cervical dilation, when labor is well-established. If at this time the woman feels no stronger uterine sensations than she is willing to accept, it is probable there will be no need for medication. Transition (the last few centimeters' dilation), the most painful time, is still ahead; but it is the shortest stage, seldom over forty-five minutes, even for a first labor. The second, expulsive stage is normally, and with proper pushing technique, the least painful part of the entire labor."

Major anesthesia is also sometimes useful, but since it carries the greatest risks and is most likely to slow labor, must be used with the most caution. The two main types of anesthesia used in vaginal deliveries are spinals and epidurals; in both, the mother is injected at the base of the spine with an agent that blocks feeling below the waist. Spinals are easier to administer but are given only just before the last contractions and, because the anesthesia is directly injected into an area rich in blood vessels, may cause a sudden drop in blood pressure as the vessels relax and the mother's blood pools. Epidurals "take" more slowly, making any side effects, including blood pressure changes, easier to manage. They are usually given earlier in labor but, because they diminish the force of contractions, often slow labor progress. (If a woman has an episiotomy and needs a shot of local anesthetic, it will not halt labor, which is almost over in any case.)

Dr. Michelle Copeland, a New York surgeon, is an example of a mother who used anesthesia wisely. Although she had planned for her first baby, Robert, to be born with as little intervention as possible, when it became clear that she was facing both a big baby and a slow labor, she decided to have an epidural in early labor "in small doses so that it would wear off in time and not interfere with the pushing. I think saving myself some pain in the beginning helped me to persevere," she adds. "The second stage lasted three and a half hours, and it was absolute agony—the baby's head had to mold considerably to get out. Although I deal with other people's pain every day, nothing had prepared me for that, and I think many women would have justifiably given up. But, being a doctor myself, I also well understand the risks of a Cesarean and I decided to continue as long as the baby wasn't in distress. I do, however, think my extra knowledge as a doctor helped me. I trusted the people I had chosen to administer the anesthesia correctly, and when forceps were needed later, I trusted my obstetrician with a difficult vaginal delivery."

What is a reasonable anesthesia use? Dublin Maternity, with its very low Cesarean rate, has curtailed the use of epidurals to only 13 per 1,000 deliveries, while in the United States many hospitals use anesthesia for one-quarter to one-half of their deliveries. "Classically, epidurals stop labor," says Dr. Haverkamp. "I don't care what it says in the textbooks. Maybe in the very, very best hands an epidural is okay, but anybody practicing obstetrics will tell you they've seen this happen over and over again. You're just crazy to interfere like that if the mother is otherwise healthy."

Walking, Liquids and the Toilet

There are several simple and natural ways to keep labor progressing and control pain. Walking is the easiest and most helpful. Childbirth educators also suggest changing position frequently. After the baby's head has engaged in the second stage, squatting, which enlarges the pelvic opening, can be very comfortable and can shorten the end of labor. If the mother begins to feel exhausted, she should by all means rest, but rather than lying flat, which slows labor, try being plumped up with pillows. Or she may want to take a warm shower, or a bath (if the membranes haven't yet ruptured), or simply put warm compresses on her abdomen. Many women don't know that they can stimulate labor with slight pinches to the nipples, which encourages natural production of oxytocin, the hormone of labor. Always, the warm, encouraging support of a relative or friend is reassuring and helps to keep labor going. When women have a "support person" nearby during labor, their need for painkillers demonstrably decreases.

Dr. Friedman, in his research on dysfunctional labor, suggested that if the descent of the baby slows in the second stage the best way to get labor going again "includes detailed attention to nutrition, fluid requirements and electrolyte imbalances." The odds, however, that a mother will be able to pay "detailed attention" to nutrition in an American hospital are about zero. Most hospitals forbid a woman to eat during labor from fear that should she need general anesthesia, she might vomit and possibly die from inhaling the stomach contents. Since, after several hours of labor, a woman will be exhausted and in a state of semistarvation, it is a rule that causes incredible discomfort but may not really provide extra protection. When a mother doesn't eat during labor, her stomach doesn't empty; what gathers there is gastric acid. Although improvements in anesthesia technique since the "empty stomach" rule was made have made fatal gagging a rare event, the British have concluded that nearly all mothers who die from general anesthesia during Cesarean section gag on this accumulated gastric acid.

The North Central Bronx obstetrics department, believing that good nutrition assisted good labor, did permit mothers to eat for the first five years it was in operation. With two thousand mothers a year, there was not a single problem. But the anesthesia department finally won in insisting on no food, although juice, milk, and other liquids are still allowed. For the most part, hospitals seem only to permit eating when mothers use alternative birth rooms—and have signed releases taking legal responsibility for bypassing the standard medical strictures of birth. Occasionally, even though the hospital will decline the legal responsibility of serving the mother food, the staff will not interfere should she bring a snack with her.

Most mothers do not seem to want much solid food during labor; childbirth educators often suggest light but nourishing snacks such as chicken broth, milk, or juice. Even water is beneficial; although it does not replenish energy, water does help conserve it. For every 5 percent of water loss through perspiration, the body loses 20 percent of its physical stamina—and labor often requires as much stamina as running a marathon. Some hospitals are so rigid that they may forbid you even to drink water; they may say you have to suck on ice chips if you feel thirsty. Silly as you may feel, suck on as many ice chips as you can.

"Another vastly overlooked aid to labor is the toilet," Diony Young says enthusiastically. "It may not be aesthetic, but you should urinate every hour anyway simply because a full bladder interferes with labor. Also, a toilet is an ideal height for a laboring position and, psychologically, it's associated with the message of letting go. Stay in there awhile and let your partner give you a nice massage."

Calcium is known to soothe pain and is considered an ideal natural aid to labor. "My advice to expectant mothers," the late nutritionist Adelle Davis wrote, "has long been to take, as soon as labor starts, a capsule containing Vitamin D and two or three calcium tablets every hour (the Vitamin D aids calcium absorption) until they are wheeled into the delivery room." Calcium, interestingly, aside from relieving pain, assists blood clotting, another helpful trait during birth (unlike aspirin, which promotes bleeding). Calcium is also important for maintaining muscle tone and strong muscular contractions.

Speaking Up

To keep your labor progressing nicely it is important to speak up, and keep hospital intrusions to a minimum. Your husband or labor coach can be very helpful here. Hospital personnel, unfortunately, tend to forget that many women have never been hospitalized before the birth of a child and that what is "routine" for the medical staff may be frightening to new mothers. If you have never used a bedpan, you may feel tense about doing so in a room where other people are present. Too frequent vaginal examinations by residents, by nurses, and by, it may begin to seem, everyone in white who walks down the hallway may be an affront to a mother's sense of modesty and leave her tense and unhappy. If these problems occur during your labor, speak up, or let your coach speak up while you protect your tranquillity and concentration. Tell hospital personnel how many times you have been examined already and ask why another is needed, or say that you wish to use the toilet, not the bedpan. Hospitals may simply lose track of the intensity of intrusions on a mother, yet creating as tranquil an atmosphere as possible is important to labor. At North Central Bronx, mothers not experiencing medical difficulties usually have only three internal examinations while they are in labor.

In short, a good, basic knowledge of labor, from methods of prepared childbirth to the proper use of medication, can only stand you in good stead, helping you both to control your own labor and prevent unnecessary medical instrusions. When you don't understand what is happening or what the hospital staff is recommending, just ask. "What is that medication or procedure? Do I really need it now? What would happen if we just waited instead and saw whether the labor proceeded naturally?"

Changing Doctors at the Last Minute

No matter how careful a woman is in choosing a doctor, or how knowledgeable she is about labor before choosing, she may come to the realization late in pregnancy that the doctor simply doesn't share her views toward birth—especially natural birth—or is incompatible in other respects. This can be entirely depressing. The mother will wonder how she could have chosen wrongly, whether all her preparation was for nothing, and whether she can possibly manage to start interviewing doctors again or make a last-minute change. It can be done, however, and it is worth doing. You will be glad in the end that you persevered.

Anne Strickland Squadron is an example. She had done considerable volunteer work for the Childbearing Center, was on its board of directors, had clear views about what she wanted for her first delivery, and looked carefully for her doctor; but eight months into her pregnancy, she realized that one doctor in the group she had chosen vehemently opposed natural birth. She did not wish to chance that he would be on duty the day her infant was born. "It was very traumatic," she recalls, "but I just left and quickly found another doctor who really was helpful. Still, I had to have my husband call to transfer my records and say I was definitely leaving. I couldn't deal with it at the time."

Esther Zorn, the Cesarean Prevention Movement leader, had the possibly more traumatic experience of having her doctor reject her. You will recall she had a Cesarean for her first baby, and for her second, in 1981, she chose a doctor who agreed to try a vaginal delivery. Since the doctor was a woman and it would be her own first vaginal delivery of a previous Cesarean mother, it seemed to be a case of women marching forward together. But when Esther was eight and a half months pregnant, the doctor said she had decided a vaginal delivery was too experimental and she couldn't agree to it. "I was surprised that I felt really free when I walked out of there," Esther Zorn comments. "If she didn't believe in it anyway, what was I doing with her?" Within two weeks, Esther Zorn had another doctor and a vaginal delivery.

Occasionally, however, another physician may not be available and the mother will have to continue where she is. In that case, Colleen Shetland suggests in the *Cesarean Prevention Clarion* that "a low profile" rather than "exposing yourself to conflicts and arguments which will only drain your energy" may be the best approach. "Do avoid as many tests as you can," she adds. "Avoid asking your doctor questions which may open areas of conflict. Associate with people who believe in what you're doing. You may choose to stay home for most of your labor. Have people with you who are informed and experienced [and] only when you feel your labor has progressed to the point it will probably not stop is it time to consider going to the hospital."

Your Own Labor Coach at Home

For women who live in communities where there isn't much choice of hospitals or attendants, or who aren't satisfied with the Cesarean rate of the available facilities—or who simply want their labor to be as tranquil as possible—there is another option. Consider hiring an obstetric nurse or other trained "labor support" person to stay with you at home through the start of labor and then accompany you to the hospital. Often, childbirth activist groups which have screened local doctors will also have a list of obstetric nurses or childbirth educators who are happy to go to a woman's home, and then to the hospital, and coach her individually. It is hard to exaggerate the real enthusiasm and interest these nurses and coaches bring to labor. You will go through the birth process with a professional who is on your side. Also, a nurse can measure your progress—even a female obstetrician in labor cannot tell by herself how far she is dilated—and prevent you from going to the hospital too soon, where "protocols" may begin to take over.

One situation in which a home labor nurse is useful

is when a mother's membranes rupture early, before strong labor starts. In this case, a hospital may start counting hours against you the moment you arrive, and soon recommend a Cesarean. But being at home keeps you away from the infectious bacteria rampant in all hospital environments—the very reason that hospitals insist on a quick delivery one way or the other. Childbirth educators often suggest that when the membranes rupture without good contractions, the mother should stay home in bed for a day, or longer if needed. (She should not, by the way, take a bath after the membranes have ruptured, but she may take a shower.) She should inform her doctor of the situation by telephone; he may want her to take her temperature from time to time to check for infection. However, some women will feel more comfortable in such a situation if a nurse comes to the house so that they have an encouraging professional close by.

Ask Those Questions, but Be Flexible

Perhaps the best reason to ask questions is to keep from being overwhelmed by situations you didn't anticipate. As you begin to learn about the facilities in your area, be flexible and open-minded. The hospital where you would want to have brain surgery may hardly be the hospital where it is best to have a baby. Often, the best-known obstetric hospital in an area is a large, regional referral center which takes in troubled pregnancies from many surrounding towns. Because of their specialization, such hospitals may be justified in having both higher Cesarean and infant mortality rates, but if your pregnancy has proceeded normally, you may do better to avoid a regional center. Where the focus is on the pathology of pregnancy, your labor, which would be considered normal in another hospital, can easily be labeled "abnormal" if it shows even the slightest variations that occur in many uncomplicated deliveries.

Parents who ordinarily wouldn't use a public hospital should at least check out those in their area. Some are old and depressing, but others offer excellent facilities—along with their unusually good obstetrics departments. Military hospitals have also been quite successful in curbing Cesarean rates—for much the same reasons public hospitals have. The federal government, by paying for the malpractice insurance of military doctors, protects them from legal pressure; and military hospitals require second opinions for all Cesareans.

Whether you want a physician- or midwife-attended birth, the fact that a hospital employs midwives usually indicates it has a strong interest in normal labor. Birthing centers are another important alternative.

Possibly, the hospitals to regard with the most suspicion are those which at first might seem the ideal place for your baby to be born. These are smaller community and suburban hospitals—quiet, clean, friendly, well decorated and, too often, obstetric disasters. Here doctors, frequently part-owners, escape internal review; here the staff doesn't have to keep up with as basic a new procedure as scalp sampling. Perhaps from her pretty room, looking across the landscaped trees crowding her window, the mother may even glimpse her physician as he comes running in at the last minute to say, "Oh, let's do a Cesarean."

Confidence to Persevere, Confidence to Decide

But, if you have asked the five basic questions above, you can come close to guaranteeing that you will never end up with a Cesarean that is so obviously thoughtless and so clearly hasty. Let's review those questions and see how worthwhile they are and what can be gained by asking them. Simply by inquiring about a hospital's and doctor's Cesarean rates, right from the start you can avoid facilities where operations are clearly out of control. By seeking a hospital with peer review, you have taken the step many doctors consider most important to curbing unnecessary Cesareans. The availability of scalp sampling can easily halve the prospects of an unnecessary "distress" Cesarean. The presence of midwives and alternative birth rooms reflects a hospital's commitment to normal labor. Being aware of hospital protocols helps you guard against automatic procedures which, too often, lead to Cesareans.

This knowledge and foresight will allow you to persevere with normal labor, confident that the professionals around you are not going to lead you to poor decisions in the rare times of unexpected trouble.

"There isn't now—and I don't think ever will be—an absolutely scientific way to decide who needs a Cesarean," says Dr. Ranney. "There is always going to be an area where the judgment and experience of the obstetrician is the key. I believe that what it comes down to is the art of obstetrics—the consummate art."

Chapter Three

SPECIAL MOTHERS
AND
NORMAL BIRTHS

S even pounds, 19¼ inches, and perfect in every way, Antonio Lopez III was delivered by a midwife at 8:48 A.M. on a Christmas morning at North Central Bronx Hospital. His birth was uncomplicated—but unusual. Antonio's mother, Miriam Lopez, a nineteen-year-old accounting student at Baruch College, had had a Cesarean section two years earlier when her twins were born. She was now quietly astonished to have managed the normal birth, which she had wanted so much but thought she could never have. Antonio's father, a twenty-year-old cook, was ecstatic to have been his wife's labor coach and relieved that she had avoided surgery. Seeing her unconscious the first time had made him "kinda nervous" and he was convinced a natural delivery was "better for her." And for North Central Bronx's groundbreaking obstetrics department, Antonio's birth was another success in promoting normal deliveries for previous Cesarean mothers. The successful program at North Central Bronx has in fact been instrumental in forcing the American obstetrics community to reexamine whether Cesarean mothers actually do need surgery for later children.

Repeat Cesarean mothers are not alone in facing Ce-

sarean rates approaching 90 to 100 percent. At many
hospitals, both breech babies and the infants of diabetic mothers are automatically delivered by Cesarean
section.

Cesarean rates of double to triple the average are
also common for mothers with hypertension (high
blood pressure) and those who have genital herpes, for
mothers expecting twins, for older mothers, and for
both postmature and premature births. Yet, except
for hypertensive mothers and, to some extent, very premature deliveries, current Cesarean practices for these
groups may be neither safe nor wise.

In some cases, such blind dependence on Cesareans
may cause deaths of mothers and babies; certainly automatic repeat Cesareans have. In other cases, Cesareans may divert attention from better ways, including
special prenatal care and individualized obstetric management, to enhance the baby's health and chance for
survival. A few hospitals, for example, are now so
skilled in caring for diabetic mothers and postmature
pregnancies that the infants have almost normal survival rates, while Cesarean rates for the mothers have
decreased significantly.

Generally, high-risk mothers who face unusual Cesarean rates will know of their condition weeks or
months ahead of the baby's birth. They will not be
happy to realize that something is "wrong," but they
will usually have plenty of time to learn all they can
and make whatever arrangements or changes are necessary. After the first shock passes, they may be pleas-
antly surprised to discover the recent progress some
hospitals and doctors have made in treating their condition.

Let's look closely at the special circumstances which may make you a high-risk mother, and see how you may be able to circumvent unnecessary surgery—even while improving the safety of your baby's delivery.

Automatic Repeats

If you have already had a Cesarean, the odds are astoundingly high that you will be given a section for your next delivery *whether you need it or not.*

The rule "Once a Cesarean, always a Cesarean" stems from the operating techniques of the early twentieth century. The high vertical incisions of the time left large uterine scars; when these mothers attempted normal labor, in about 5 percent of cases the scar would rupture, creating a severe emergency for both mother and baby from bleeding and shock. However, with the low uterine, or "bikini," incision which has been standard for Cesareans since the 1920s, scar rupture during normal labor is so rare that there are not even good estimates of its occurrence.

Nonetheless, 200,000 women and infants a year continue to be exposed to routine surgery for the sake of a rule made half a century ago and based upon information that is not only outdated but dangerous. In 1969, for example, the British reported that infant deaths from respiratory distress syndrome, a common ailment when Cesareans are performed in the absence of labor, were 47 per 1,000 for automatic repeat Cesarean babies delivered before the start of labor, 3 per 1,000 for Cesarean babies delivered after the start of labor, and 1 per 1,000 for vaginal babies. In the intervening years, sophisticated nursery care for babies with respiratory distress has slashed these death rates; yet it is clear that automatic repeat operations have killed more infants than any other known recent medical error, including the major tragedies of thalidomide and DES.

Let's look at the largest recent study, conducted at the University of Washington and published in 1981, which compares trial labor and automatic repeat operations. After reviewing hundreds of thousands of pregnancies in Europe and the United States, doctors found a maternal death rate of 3.8 per 10,000 for women who were allowed trial labor, whether they completed a vaginal delivery or not, versus a death rate of 4.6 per 10,000 when mothers had Cesareans without any attempt at labor.

Given surgical risks, maternal deaths are not unexpected. But the real jolt was the fact that when mothers were allowed trial labor, only 119 babies per 10,000 died, but for automatic repeats with no trial labor, 158 babies per 10,000 died. The excess deaths of the automatic repeat babies, again, were almost all caused by respiratory distress.

For decades, repeat Cesarean mothers have been told that the extra risk to them guarded their babies from harm, but this is not the case. Mothers are now told that "sophisticated testing" is finally conquering respiratory distress, by enabling doctors to be certain the baby's lungs are mature even if labor hasn't yet begun. But is *this* true?

Despite advanced technology, respiratory distress, although less frequent, has proved unexpectedly stub-

born. The tests seem to fail in 3 to 4 percent of cases—
no small amount when we have 200,000 repeat Cesareans a year; moreover, automatic repeat babies some-
time develop respiratory distress even when testing
before the operation has confirmed that their lungs are,
in fact, mature. For this reason, some doctors now suspect that a form of respiratory distress called "persistent fetal circulation," which is different from the
"classic" disease of immature infants, occurs *only*
among Cesarean babies with physically mature lungs.
"Although we don't understand very well what happens or why seemingly mature infants develop distress," comments one pediatrician studying persistent
fetal circulation, "the problem evidently is not timing,
but the mode of delivery—that is, the disease is sec-
ondary to the Cesarean itself."

Respiratory Distress Versus Rupture: No Contest

All in all, then, we know that trial labor is safer for
most previous Cesarean mothers and their newborns.
In 1982, the American College of Obstetricians and
Gynecologists did finally approve trial labor at hospitals with around-the-clock blood banks and readily
available operating rooms and personnel. Yet, this still
does not mean that it will be easy for you to find a
doctor and a hospital prepared to allow trial labor. Most
hospitals seriously restrict mothers whom they permit
to try labor—they won't permit labor for women who
have medical conditions such as diabetes or hyperten-

sion, for example, or obstetric complications such as bleeding or poor fetal growth—and they also expect the mother to produce the records from her previous operation.

The reason for this is to confirm the dimensions of the uterine scar; even when a small bikini scar shows on the skin, sometimes the uterine incision underneath is vertical. Vertical incisions are usually done for reasons of medical emergency. On the other hand, some few doctors, for their own convenience, still use the easier, but uglier vertical skin incision while employing a low horizontal incision of the uterus underneath. In that case, since it is the uterine incision which is important, the mother is a candidate for trial labor.

But, aside from medical considerations, it takes a long time for hospitals to change their policies, and many hospitals still try to discourage nearly all women from trial labor. You may be told constantly of the "dangers" of scar rupture, and you may be asked to sign what birth activist Nancy Cohen describes as "Draconian consent forms so full of hypothetical risks that it's a wonder they don't scare off everyone." These consent forms are there to protect the hospital legally, and you should not let them scare you. You may also be told that it would be "a waste" for you to go through labor and then possibly still have to have a Cesarean, when it would be "so much more convenient" just to schedule the operation. In fact, at hospitals which allow trial labor, well over half of previous Cesarean mothers who try do complete a vaginal delivery, so the odds are on your side. But more important, because labor primes the fetal lungs for breathing and slashes the prospects of respiratory distress, it is hardly wasted. Even if you do have a second Cesarean, you will also have the assurance that you tried your best and that your baby benefited.

Once again, remember that there is simply no contest between the risk of respiratory distress and the risk of scar rupture. Since the rupture is confined to a small area, doctors can quickly perform an emergency Cesarean and remove the baby before hemorrhaging is fatal; infant survival is close to 100 percent, which is certainly not the case with respiratory distress. As for mothers, once again, *there is not a single recorded case in the standard medical literature of a mother's having died because her low "bikini" scar ruptured.*

The experience of North Central Bronx, Bronx Municipal, and Einstein hospitals illustrates the great safety of trial labor. In nine years of encouraging trial labor, not one of these large, busy hospitals, each with more than two thousand deliveries a year, has encountered a single full rupture of a low uterine incision. Thus Dr. Schulman is in the interesting position of having unique and long experience with trial labor, but having almost nothing to say about uterine ruptures. "The textbooks are full of elaborate advice about how to predict whether a scar will rupture. But not having seen one myself—I've seen scars stretch far without splitting—I do not have elaborate advice on the subject," he comments. "And sometimes I wonder where the textbooks get theirs."

Most Mothers Can

Can a previous Cesarean mother tell beforehand what her prospects are of having a normal birth, or V-BAC (vaginal birth after a Cesarean)? The reason for trial labor is that there is simply no better way of predicting which Cesarean mothers will complete a vaginal delivery than there is of predicting delivery outcomes for non-Cesarean mothers. However, at hospitals both in Europe and the United States, no matter what the reason for the first Cesarean, the majority of mothers selected to try labor succeed for the second delivery. In fact, if the first Cesarean was performed because of a condition which rarely occurs in another pregnancy, such as a breech or a placenta which interfered with the delivery (placenta previa), there is an 85 to 100 percent chance of completing a normal delivery next time. If the first Cesarean resulted from arrested labor, fetal distress, or "failed" oxytocin augmentation of labor, several hospitals have reported that between 65 and 80 percent of such Cesarean mothers can have normal second deliveries.

Even when the Cesarean was for disproportion, about half of the mothers complete normal deliveries. It is interesting to note that many mothers who had Cesareans for disproportion are able to deliver normally a much larger baby the second time. Despite a first Cesarean for "disproportion," X rays still cannot predict that particular mother's chance for a vaginal delivery the second time. In one major study, more previous Cesarean mothers with "abnormal" pelvic X rays delivered normally than did those with X ray confirmation of normal pelvic size and structure. Again, trying is the real test. Only when the doctor tried to induce labor the first time and failed, do the chances of a normal delivery seem to slip below 50 percent. But there is still no reason not to try; you might just go the distance.

What About Labor After Several Cesareans?

Although many hospitals limit trial labor to women with a single previous Cesarean, there is no medical reason not to try a normal delivery if you have had more than one Cesarean. At Bronx Municipal, women who have had two or three Cesareans routinely deliver vaginally. Nor does there appear to be a limit to the number of normal deliveries which can occur after a Cesarean. With the large farm families common in Yankton, Dr. Ranney, for one, has delivered as many as six later infants vaginally to a mother whose first delivery was a Cesarean. "Right from the beginning," he says, "I couldn't see, if you knew a woman was going to have four or five or six more children, giving her operations over and over again."

Actually, it will probably be some time before even the best informed doctors, hospitals, and mothers appreciate the real value of trial labor. It is important, for example, in looking at the success rate of mothers who have tried labor, to realize that many hospitals still allow only a small proportion of *all* previous Cesarean mothers to make the attempt. They refuse the rest for a variety of "medical" reasons. Probably Los Angeles Women's Hospital is the only hospital in the United States which has dropped all such restrictions and allows any woman who has had one Cesarean to try labor if she wants to. She will now be treated like any other mother; only a medical condition that would preclude labor for a non-Cesarean mother would preclude it for her. And, since many of the mothers at Women's Hospital had their surgery in Mexico and cannot obtain their records, the hospital no longer even requires a surgical history.

At Women's Hospital many previous Cesarean mothers—diabetics, women with twins, breech babies— now deliver vaginally who would be absolutely forbidden to do so at other hospitals, and 83 percent of its trial-labor mothers now complete a vaginal delivery.

This remarkable success continues to be exciting for mothers and hospital staff alike. Dr. Jeffrey Phelan recalls that when he came to Women's in 1981 he had no faith in trial labor and yet, on his first day, witnessed four successful cases. His own wife, Marilyn, had three Cesarean deliveries. "One of her real complaints about her deliveries was that she felt cheated," he relates, "and shouldn't have needed an operation all three times. After I started here, I had to go home and say to her, 'You know all those things you've been saying about Cesareans for years—you were right.'"

Enhancing Your Success

Because policies about trial labor differ so widely, it is especially important to find the right doctor and hospital. Probably less than half of American obstetricians now attempt trial labor in their practices at all, and while some hospitals, because of patient demand, seem to encourage the procedure, they can be almost punitive toward the mothers. In an outrageous twist on payment practices, one hospital in Montana demands that trial-labor mothers pay the full cost of keeping an operating room on call all the time they are in labor. But hospitals do not demand that any other patients who might require emergency surgery pay for an operating room unless they do in fact use one. Watch for such signs of hostility toward previous Cesarean mothers.

In general, the longer hospitals have encouraged trial labor, giving their staff time to develop enthusiasm about the procedure, the greater the prospects of success for the individual mother become. However, there is no predictable pattern to finding doctors or hospitals enthusiastic about trial labor; in Wichita, Kansas, all four hospitals with obstetric services now permit trial labor, while women who live in the outlying towns can rarely arrange for trial labor at smaller, rural hospitals. On the other hand, the Wisconsin State Cesarean Prevention Movement has reported that V-BACs are very hard to obtain in Madison, a major university city, while about forty miles away, in the outlying Janesville-Delevan area, there are both doctors and hospitals quite willing to attempt trial labor. You might assume too that younger doctors would change the fastest; but often older doctors, with their greater confidence in their own common sense, are the most willing to proceed with V-BACs. If you cannot find a cooperative doctor on your own, look for a nearby birth activist organization. The Cesarean Prevention Movement is expanding rapidly and has referral lists of doctors who perform V-BACs (see Appendix). If you have a choice, you should also check what percentage of previous Cesarean mothers the hospital delivers normally. Other things being equal, you would clearly want the hospital which offered the greatest prospect for normal birth.

Many women who have had a previous Cesarean will need a little extra encouragement when they try labor for a subsequent delivery. They will need plenty of warm support from their doctors and hospital staff; they will also need time. For previous Cesarean mothers who didn't labor at all the first time, this will be their first labor, and those whose labor was cut short can expect a longer-than-average second labor. Birth activist Nancy Cohen, for instance, reports that among 105 successful V-BACs she has coached, active labor continued as long as forty-four hours (though also as short as forty-five minutes).

Women will also want to review their own attitudes toward V-BAC. If, after being fully informed of the benefits, a woman is uncomfortable about attempting a vaginal birth, the final decision is of course up to her. Dr. Samuel Oberlander, the first director of obstetrics at North Central Bronx, was astonished when he returned to private practice in suburban Westchester County, to encounter some previous Cesarean mothers who had no interest in trial labor. Accustomed as he was to the enthusiasm for trial labor which had communicated itself so easily to mothers at North Central, their fear mystified him. "I still don't know quite what bothers them," he comments. "Maybe a deep-seated fear of the scar rupturing; or maybe they see the Cesarean as just a means of getting the birth out of the way. I don't really know. The midwives back at North Central say I should sit these women down and talk them into it. But, in my experience, it doesn't really work to talk a woman into trial labor. When she is nervous or reluctant, she usually ends up with a Cesarean anyway."

Do be certain, however, that if you decide against a V-BAC, it is truly a choice and not a sense of discouragement about normal birth. Probably the best thing to do if you are uncertain is talk to another Cesarean mother who has had a successful V-BAC. You may be interested to learn that she had the same fears you might have and yet—she still had a normal birth!

Your Own Nurse

In a provocative insight into the conditions of normal delivery, McMaster University Medical Center in Ontario, Canada, has reported that no matter what a mother's reason for a previous Cesarean, if she arrived at the hospital more than 3 centimeters dilated, she had a 67 percent chance of finishing her delivery normally; with less than 3 centimeters dilation, the chances were much smaller. We aren't sure why this disparity exists —it could be that mothers who are well dilated are simply in good labor; but it could also be that the hospital environment impinges itself on previous Cesarean mothers, nervous as they may be from a past operation, and slows their labor. Previous Cesarean mothers may be advised to come to the hospital for observation as soon as labor begins, whereas other mothers are told to stay home as long as possible. Yet some childbirth educators feel that previous Cesarean mothers will benefit most from the relaxed atmosphere at home and advise them to consider hiring an obstetric nurse to stay with them there until labor is well established—and then at the hospital, throughout the delivery. The value of this kind of personal support has been more than apparent in the experience of Nancy Cohen. Of the previous Cesarean mothers she has personally coached and counseled, 91 percent have had successful vaginal deliveries.

If you would like to try this approach, first discuss these points with your doctor and make sure the hospital will allow your coach into the delivery room. Sometimes there is opposition and sometimes there isn't. Lindy Johnson is a Berkeley, California, obstetric nurse who, having had a V-BAC herself, is particularly interested in assisting previous Cesarean mothers. With an associate, she has started a service called Labor of Love, which supplies personal nurses for labor support. "Usually, when they know you're a nurse, they're glad to see you at the hospital and there's no trouble about staying right with the mother," she says. Equally important, part of this service is to provide nursing help to keep the mothers safely at home until they are in good labor. "Hospital environments do impede labor," Ms. Johnson adds, "and hospitals are impatient by nature."

Why Doctors Get Furious

But, for most women, the doctor's opposition to trial labor—and not their own fears or the hospital environment—will prove the largest hurdle to a successful V-BAC. You may, in fact, be astonished by the outright fury that the suggestion of trial labor still sometimes raises. What you must remember—in fairness to the doctor, but equally to protect yourself from being discouraged—is that most doctors were taught again and again that trial labor is mortally dangerous. Even though the information is outdated, it takes time for obstetricians to accept that. As a young doctor now doing postgraduate work in perinatology at Bronx Municipal Hospital explains, "I was originally taught to think catastrophe if a Cesarean mother labors. At Bronx Municipal, trial labors have been the philosophy for so long it begins to seem normal. But, I can tell you that if you don't have the experience, at first you are afraid. Just that one thought—'catastrophe, catastrophe'— keeps going through your mind. It took some months, actually, for me to get over it, but after eighteen months here, I've never seen a catastrophic situation from trial labor and now I think, 'Let's give the lady a real chance.' "

In these circumstances, you will obviously have to prepare yourself mentally to persevere against the opposition to trial labor. If most women in the United States can now find at least one doctor or hospital within driving distance that "allows" V-BACs, they still won't necessarily find an ideal atmosphere. Recall the case of Esther Zorn, whose doctor said she was willing to attempt a V-BAC and then abruptly announced, when Ms. Zorn was eight and a half months pregnant, that she had decided trial labor was "too experimental." Esther Zorn did find another obstetrician who approved trial labor, but she went into labor a week early when he was out of town. His partner reluctantly consented to deliver her vaginally, after making his disapproval plain. Ms. Zorn took two obstetric nurses with her as labor coaches and the delivery was a success, but the atmosphere was full of tension and acrimony. "He gave me an episiotomy from here to Kansas, which was sewn up so badly that I later had to have three sessions of cryo-surgery to correct it," she relates. "And don't think I don't think his anger at me didn't have something to do with that." Nonetheless, she certainly preferred a normal birth, no matter how grudgingly offered, to an automatic operation.

But trial labor can also be an occasion when you join with a doctor at a profound, inspiring level. Many doctors, after all, regard trial labor as a major reform in obstetric practice and relish pioneering it with their patients. Even twenty years ago, Josephine Williams, a Brooklyn mother who decided she simply did not want another Cesarean for her second delivery, was fortunate to find excellent medical support. She and her husband "thought the best way to deal with it was to go straight to the top." They approached Dr. Elmer Kramer, a prominent obstetrician at New York Hospital. "He accepted me as his patient and I accepted him as my doctor on this basis," Ms. Williams recalls. "My labor started very slowly. I was in the hospital for a day. The residents had me walking and everything, but nothing worked. Finally, Dr. Kramer said he'd have to operate. I begged him to try just one more thing. He gave me Pitocin. [Using Pitocin after a previous Cesarean is controversial, and opinion is divided among doctors who will use it and those who won't.] I found I could control the contractions very well. Jonathan is now six foot three and hale and hearty and talented in every way, and was I ever glad that I didn't have to go home feeling the way I had felt after a section."

Breech Babies

Nearly all breech babies are delivered by Cesarean section in the United States, accounting for 90,000 Cesareans each year. Many hospitals will not deliver any breech baby vaginally. At a symposium in California a few years ago, some doctors stated quite candidly that no matter what the evidence favoring vaginal delivery for some breech infants, the malpractice situation virtually precluded them from considering anything but Cesareans for these sometimes difficult births. Nonetheless, scrupulous research shows that vaginal delivery of a full-term breech baby is sometimes safer and easier. If your baby is in a breech position, keep in mind that it may turn on its own up until the last moment, but you must also begin to consider the alternatives.

Breech babies occur in about 4 percent of all births, and 6 percent of first births. Because more babies turn spontaneously toward the end of pregnancy, the breech rate increases with prematurity; at, say, twenty-five weeks, about 15 percent of babies are breech. A few breech babies will slip undiscovered past even the best obstetricians, but most of the time the obstetrician, simply by external examination, will discover well before the delivery that the baby hasn't turned.

Breech babies assume several positions. Most are frank breech babies with buttocks down and legs pointing up; some are complete breeches with buttocks down and the legs crooked against the body; and others, footling breeches, will extend one or both legs down the birth canal first. The baby's head can be in a flexed position—tucked downward toward the chest—which is best for birth; a military position, or facing forward; or hyperextended, flung backward as though looking toward the sky (sometimes called "stargazing babies"). Your baby's position, usually confirmed by X ray, will influence its delivery. Frank breeches with flexed heads are the best candidates for vaginal delivery. With complete and footling breeches, there is an increased chance that the umbilical cord can slip around the baby to exit first, threatening the fetal oxygen supply. If the baby's head is not flexed, there is an increased danger of the head's becoming stuck going through the pelvis. It is then too late to resort to a Cesarean.

Transverse-lie babies are another group of malpositioned infants; they lie curled across the bottom of the uterus as though taking a nap on a couch. Although these babies are rare, because one shoulder descends first into the birth canal, completely blocking the baby's exit, they invariably require a Cesarean.

Risks for Mothers and Babies

Studies have shown no overall improvement in survival for normal-weight frank breeches as Cesarean rates have climbed; evidently, at the rates of a decade ago, doctors were already catching all such babies who might have become fatally stuck during a breech birth. However, another worry about the vaginal delivery of breech babies is that there could be trauma to the head, causing brain damage. But considerable evidence indicates that a vaginal delivery is no more likely to cause brain damage for normal-weight breeches than a Cesarean.

The Royal Victoria Hospital, in reviewing all deliveries of normal-weight frank breech babies over a period of fifteen years, focused on the brain damage question. Doctors there compared various signs of possible damage for the years 1963 to 1973, when the breech Cesarean rate was 22 percent, and the years 1978–79, when the breech Cesarean rate had zoomed to 94 percent. Despite this inordinate change in birth method (and despite the monitoring, sonar, and other tools of fetal assessment available in the later years), the rate of asphyxia, or severe oxygen deprivation, stayed at 17 percent for all normal-weight frank breech newborns in both periods. The incidence of obvious central-nervous-system trauma remained at 1 percent in both periods. So a 400 percent increase in the Cesarean rate had not resulted in even a 1 percent reduction in conditions which might indicate brain damage.

There have also been large follow-up studies comparing the intellectual performance of breech babies who were born by Cesarean and those born vaginally. While such studies disagree on some points—as studies will—massive and carefully constructed research shows that vaginally delivered full-term breeches are just like other children as they reach school age. Dr. Edward Quilligan, the former chief of obstetrics at Los Angeles Women's Hospital, has made a special point of studying breeches, and states flatly that there is not a single well-done study which suggests that normal weight frank breeches delivered vaginally develop more neurological or intellectual handicaps than those delivered by Cesarean.

Shoulder dislocations, or Erb's palsy, are sometimes a hazard in vaginal breech births, although shoulder dislocations also occasionally occur when breech infants are delivered by Cesarean. Once again, Cesareans are not magic; either way, extra skill is needed to manipulate a breech baby. While most of these dislocations heal within weeks, sometimes the baby's arm is permanently weakened. Shoulder dislocations can be avoided if the doctor doesn't try to pull out the baby too fast; therefore it is crucial with breech deliveries to find doctors or midwives who know what they are doing. North Central Bronx, for example, which still delivers well over half its breeches normally, rarely has a case of Erb's palsy. "What we do," explains Theresa Dondero, "when the shoulder seems stuck is let the birth proceed at its own pace instead of pulling at the baby. Then the shoulder just drops out."

In short, documented problems with frank breech babies delivered vaginally are rare when the attendant is skilled and knowledgeable. But breech Cesareans still pose all the usual risks of surgery.

Los Angeles Women's Hospital has done what seems to be the only study to define risks to both mothers and infants from breech deliveries. The hospital randomly assigned mothers of normal-weight frank breeches to be delivered either vaginally or by Cesarean. Half the mothers in the Cesarean group developed fever and infections—in two cases so severely that they required hysterectomies, thereby ending their ability to have children at all. Two of fifty-five vaginally delivered infants did sustain shoulder dislocations when doctors pulled them out a little too fast; while their arms mended well, this again was a warning that physicians who conduct vaginal breech deliveries must be experienced. Only one infant in each group had a low Apgar score, and the only deaths were caused by severe birth defects unrelated to the delivery method.

"I think," says Dr. Quilligan, "that the value of this study is we can give the mothers some real data to help with their decisions. There's no mathematic formula for judging these things, but I do think the past decade has shifted a little too far toward trying to get 'perfect babies.' That's partly why the Cesarean rate for breech has gone so high. I would like to see the mother balanced back in a little, and certainly there's nothing that supports doing Cesareans for all breeches."

And, another random study at Women's Hospital since then has suggested that, with proper selection, perhaps half of nonfrank—that is, footling and complete—breeches can be delivered vaginally with impressive safety.

Nonetheless, you may find it almost impossible to locate a doctor willing to attempt a vaginal delivery of a breech infant. In the first place, obstetricians trained in the past five to ten years have usually received so little instruction in the normal delivery of breeches that they are not adequately prepared. But even for trained doctors, the issue has become so volatile that common sense has gone by the wayside. Some doctors, for reasons that defy logic, will try for a vaginal delivery only when the mother has already delivered a previous child vaginally, a dictum presumably based on the mother's having "proven" her capacity for vaginal birth. But, for reasons not understood, prolapse of the umbilical cord occurs less often in first births which happen to be breech than in later ones. Also, later babies tend to be larger than first babies, another potential problem during breech delivery. All in all, the first-time breech mother is statistically a better candidate for normal delivery.

Older doctors who trained when most breeches were delivered vaginally and who have faith in their own common sense may be your best bet if you are expecting a breech birth. Also, midwives are now often better trained in the normal delivery of breech infants than many obstetricians. In fact, in some localities, midwives may be the only attendants willing to do a vaginal delivery. Jeanne Fauci, whose daughter Tai was delivered at Roosevelt Hospital, the first private hospital in Manhattan where midwives could have their own practices, found plenty of reassurance right from the start. "Immediately when we knew she was a breech, the midwives told me they would make every effort to see I had a normal delivery, and that gave me a lot of confidence in myself," she recalls. "Then, what was interesting, at the delivery, we were asked if some interns who had never seen a normal breech birth could come watch. I said, 'Sure, if it's going to help their education or training.' I didn't care. My husband and I were just glad that we could get this chance."

What You Can Do to Help the Birth Along

There are two interesting strategies mothers can use to promote successful vaginal deliveries for breech babies. The first, visualization, is increasingly popular and should not be dismissed out of hand. It is simply the power of positive thinking, reinforced by imagination. You relax several times a day and imagine a pleasant, positive birth scene; visualize your baby—head first or bottom first—making steady progress down the birth canal. Put a nice smile on its face! Visualization will help in all births, but is especially effective in difficult ones, so practice this again and again to dispel worry. You might be amazed at the results when you turn your mind frequently to this happy picture.

The second has to do with your position during birth. Some childbirth educators recommend a standing squat position as the best for breech delivery. In this position you stand, with someone behind you holding you under the arms for support, and squat slightly from the knees with your legs apart, somewhat like a ballerina doing pliés. The advantage, Dr. Michael Odent, a French obstetrician, has written, is that "as soon as the breech is delivered, the whole body comes," thereby eliminating the delay between the deliveries of the buttocks and the head which occurs when you lie flat on a delivery table.

You will want to discuss your position with your doctor beforehand, and practice the standing squat with your labor coach under your doctor's supervision in preparation for the birth.

Turning a Breech

But you may be able to avoid the breech dilemma altogether by having your doctor turn the baby. To look at the overwhelming advantages of this alternative, let's go back to South Dakota and Dr. Ranney.

When he first began to turn breeches, Dr. Ranney was not as concerned about Cesarean section as he was about the health risks and higher death rates of breech babies no matter how they were delivered. He recalls vividly when he first became concerned about breech births. "It was 1949, a year after I came to Yankton as the area's first obstetrician," he says. "It was the mother's first baby, and she was of healthy, hearty Dutch stock. Everything was proceeding just fine when the cord prolapsed. It was an extreme emergency and I ended up doing a forceps delivery with the forceps actually inside the cervix, something that's almost never done. We got a good baby, but that incident set me thinking. Personally, I don't mind doing a breech delivery. I feel I can get an average size baby through an average size pelvis as safely backward or forward, although I couldn't say that of today's residents. As for a difficult breech—what are the most interesting events in life? The ones that call on all your skills and concentration. For me, getting a good baby after a difficult breech is a thrill unlike any other in obstetrics. But I'm not here to be thrilled. I'm here to help the patients, and I decided to find out what I could do to avoid breech deliveries whenever possible.

"So I went back to the textbooks and used some common sense and decided to attempt external versions on breech babies." From the first, his success with version —the procedure takes him only one to five minutes— led him to use it for nearly all breech and transverse-lie babies in his care. Because the fetus, being smaller and well surrounded by amniotic fluid, turns more easily well before term, Dr. Ranney elected to perform most versions between the thirtieth and thirty-second week of pregnancy, even though some of the babies could still be expected to turn themselves spontaneously.

In summarizing twenty-one years' experience with version in *The American Journal of Obstetrics and Gynecology,* he noted that he was successful in turning 90.9 percent of babies on whom he attempted version, and that in his practice only .6 percent of babies are still malpositioned at delivery, versus the usual 4 percent. Only 6 percent of the turned breeches were finally delivered by Cesarean, while 21 percent of the breeches he was not able to turn had to be delivered by Cesarean section. You can well imagine how phenomenal the savings in surgery would be at hospitals where the breech Cesarean rate has reached 90 or 100 percent.

Nonetheless, the real triumph of version was not the savings in Cesarean deliveries, but the condition of the babies. Breech babies tend to be premature, but the prematurity rate of Dr. Ranney's turned breeches fell from the usual 20 to 30 percent to only 3 percent! Along with this decline in prematurity, neonatal mortality for the turned babies dropped to one-third that for overall neonatal deaths in Ranney's practice. Dr. Ranney can't fully explain the reduced prematurity among turned breeches, but he suggests that when an unturned baby's legs remain in the lower womb, its ordinary kicking may stimulate the uterus into premature labor. Although a Danish obstetrician has also reported that turned breeches at his hospitals have one-third the mortality rate of non-turned breeches, no one else seems to have specifically studied the question of version and prematurity. "I know these numbers are right for my population," Dr. Ranney adds, "but I'm also old enough to know you sometimes get effects in one population that you don't in another. I only wish someone else would set up a study and try and replicate this to see if I'm correct that version may finally be the answer for the premature breech."

Version Technique and Timing

You may wonder how this one-to-five-minute somersault, with its wonderful results, is accomplished. In fact, the procedure is very simple. The mother empties her bladder, then lies on her back, relaxed, with her thighs slightly flexed. The obstetrician places one hand on the mother's abdomen under the location of the baby's buttocks and one behind its head, and carefully pushes the baby around until its head is below its buttocks; at that point, the doctor quickly shifts hands and completes pressing the head toward the pelvic inlet. Very occasionally, the doctor may need to insert his fingers up the vagina to dislodge a fetus wedged deep in the pelvis. Dr. Ranney emphasizes that the physician's attitude is as important as technique. "The brains, nerves, muscles and fingers of the obstetrician should be sensitively elastic," he has written. "This is no place for a hasty or domineering approach, which is futile, and possibly dangerous. If the fetus will not be turned forward, it may be turned backward. If not today, then probably at the next office visit. With experience, one learns to be gently persistent within reasonable physiologic limits, almost coaxing the fetus around and never exceeding safe limits of pressure or tension.

"This is a gentle art," he adds. "And I mean 'gentle.' I don't know how you really teach this to someone. A good obstetrician will pick it up in two or three demonstrations, but others just can't learn it."

As with trial labor, version is relatively new in this country, and guidelines for doing it are not well established. Dr. Ranney performs versions in his clinic office, using only a stethoscope to check on the fetus; but many doctors consider this a hospital outpatient procedure, do a sonogram in advance, and monitor the fetus electronically during version. Some give the mother drugs to relax the uterus.* Dr. Ranney will turn almost any single breech baby except when the mother has a history of bleeding, a classical Cesarean scar, or ruptured membranes. Other doctors won't turn a variety of mothers, including those with hypertension, diabetes, or any Cesarean scar.

The main argument about version, however, has to do with timing. Dr. Ranney believes first babies should be turned by the thirty-second week of gestation, or about eight weeks before most pregnancies reach term, and later babies by the thirty-fourth week. He prefers to turn babies early to avoid prematurity and because version is easier when the baby is smaller. However, about 30 percent of babies turned early will turn themselves right back to breech and may need two or more versions. "One pertinacious fetus," Ranney wrote, "required eight external versions before he retained the vertex position." On the other hand, at Los Angeles Women's Hospital, versions are done at thirty-seven to thirty-nine weeks—a schedule evidently favored by most hospitals now performing version—and no fetus has yet turned itself back to a breech position. The

* The same drugs, used to relax the uterus over periods of weeks or even months to prevent premature labor, occasionally have unexpected consequences for the mother; their brief use during version is probably much safer, but has not been studied closely.

success rate at Women's Hospital, however, is about 70 percent—compared with Dr. Ranney's 90 percent, evidently the highest ever reported in the United States or Europe.

Even though version is such a simple procedure, you may be hard pressed to find a doctor to turn your baby. The continuing opposition to version may seem even more surprising than opposition to V-BACs, but the fact is some doctors have had little success at what seems so tantalizingly easy. If the medical literature contains success stories about version, it also contains reports from physicians who managed to turn so few babies that the procedure was not worth their time. Once again, the confidence and enthusiasm of the physician are crucial. "I would say," comments Dr. Jeffrey Phelan, director of the External Version Clinic at Los Angeles Women's Hospital, "that it took me some months to feel comfortable about version. Once you get your fears out of the way, though, version is really—Well, it's fun! The mothers readily accept it; they don't want Cesareans. Very few have ever refused. And since we've never had any side effects requiring intervention, the doctors are getting comfortable, too."

As a substitute for version, some childbirth educators believe that exercise can help in turning a baby, although others doubt it. Valmai Elkins, a childbirth educator at the McGill University School of Physical and Occupational Therapy in Montreal, believes strongly in the potential of exercise. She recommends mothers use the "knee-chest" position taught in most childbirth education classes to relieve backache. If you want to try, be sure you have your doctor's approval, and then

ask her or an instructor to show you the precise position. If you do this exercise for fifteen minutes every
two hours during the day, evidently babies who are
going to turn will do so within five days. Another exercise is to lie down for ten minutes, twice a day, using
pillows to raise your pelvis nine to twelve inches
higher than your head. This exercise may be done for
weeks and should be started by about the thirtieth to
thirty-sixth week of pregnancy.

The search for a willing doctor, however, is clearly
the best course. If you can't find a doctor nearby who
performs version, try calling the nearest medical school
on the off chance that a version program has been
started there. Doctors trained in Europe are also a good
prospect, because the technique is commonplace
there. "Oh, yes, I used to do this all the time," comments a European-trained doctor now affiliated with
one of the most expensive hospitals in New York City.
"But here, the hospital doesn't want us to do it. Don't
ask me why, because I don't know."

Dr. Ranney, however, does not suggest you call him.
"Women telephone from all over the country who want
to fly to Yankton for a version, but I won't do it. Aside
from the fact I don't think women should be on air-
planes in late pregnancy, you see, I know my patients
well. They're very relaxed and I've followed their history closely. I think that does account for some of my
success. I don't know that I'd get the same results with
strangers.

"You know," he adds, "sometimes people ask me,
'How the devil could you stay in Yankton for thirty-five
years?' But, being in a small town, where people trust

you, you can practice medicine in a different way. I think I've been lucky. It's given me opportunities I don't think doctors really get anymore."

Overdue Babies

Pregnancy usually lasts about forty weeks, although a few weeks' variation one way or the other is perfectly normal. If, however, your pregnancy stretches longer than forty-two weeks, counting from the last menstrual period, your baby will be considered "postmature." About 10 percent of pregnancies are classified as postmature, although many women have simply miscalculated their menstrual dates. Cesarean rates for postmature pregnancies have reached 50 percent, partly because doctors try to induce labor, without success. Unfortunately, induction can often be a wasted effort for a baby that would, in any case, have appeared at its "proper" time, a few days later, or, occasionally, cause a premature birth, with the resulting problems. Yet, when the fetus truly is postmature, the placenta may start to deteriorate and the infant become dangerously malnourished.

How can real postdates be distinguished from "premature" postdates? In the past few years, Women's Hospital has learned to treat overdue pregnancies in a way that has brought survival for the babies almost to the hospital average for normal, full-term pregnancies, while at the same time cutting the Cesarean rate of mothers by half.

Diagnostic Tests and Caution

"Postdate" explains Dr. Sze-Ya Yeh, the director of
the Women's Hospital Post-Date Clinic, "is a definition
of chronological time. This is different from saying the
biological function of the placenta has started to deteriorate. After all, there is a normal variation for the
length of healthy pregnancies. Here we have roughly
10 percent who go beyond forty-two weeks; but only 3
percent will go beyond forty-three weeks and less than
1 percent beyond 44 weeks. Now, the textbooks absolutely say you can't let a pregnancy go beyond forty-
four weeks, and many doctors will intervene before
then, but we still believe in nature. What we try to do
is detect the biological phenomenon—if the baby is
really threatened. No test is perfect, but with combined
tests, you can do very well."

Here is where the new obstetrical diagnostic and
monitoring equipment can be used, not as an intrusion,
but to point the path toward a normal delivery. At the
Post-Date Clinic, mothers are given estriol tests—estriol is a hormone whose concentration in the blood
should rise toward the end of pregnancy; "non-stress"
tests, in which the baby's heart rhythms are watched
on an electronic monitor; and "contraction stress" tests,
which involve inducing brief contractions and watch-
ing the baby's heart patterns as it responds to this stim-
ulus. Rather belatedly, doctors have realized they can
often induce contractions simply by stimulating the
mother's nipples so she produces internal oxytocin, the

necessary hormone, rather than by administering oxytocin intravenously as used to be done.

The rule at Women's Hospital is to proceed conservatively. Mothers who don't have well-documented
menstrual dates are never artificially induced unless
they have had poor results on both the non-stress and
contraction stress tests. Among the first 880 postdate
mothers treated with these procedures, there were
only eight perinatal deaths—three from severe abnormalities and five babies of mothers who had not come
routinely for their tests. With the clinic's "conservative
approach and strict criteria for induction," the Cesarean rate for postterm mothers dropped to 15.8 percent,
very close to the hospital's overall 12 percent rate.

"I think the pressure of our large population helps
get changes in treatment here," Dr. Yeh says. "People
will try another way because they're solving large
problems. For us, you're talking about five hundred
Cesareans a year, so it's a major challenge to manage
this population well. For a private doctor, it's a few
Cesareans a year in his own practice and he may not
have the same incentive to think about it. Also, there is
the problem of testing. Most private doctors don't have
a lab where they can get back an estriol reading in
twenty-four hours, which is necessary for our plan.
However, estriol has some problems of accuracy, and I
would say general opinion is moving toward the contraction stress test as the critical one for the postdate.
Private doctors still can't do that because they usually
don't have a monitor in their office. But they could
send the patient to a hospital for the monitoring. The
only thing is, you have to be sure of your personnel.

We rely on the nursing staff at Women's Hospital to screen the postdates and they are very good at it."

Keep in mind that the percentage of women who forget their menstrual dates is about the same in private hospitals and clinics alike, so if your pregnancy is overdue, chances are you have simply confused or forgotten your dates. But, as Dr. Yeh points out, if you are a private patient, it may be more difficult for you to find a doctor who will monitor you closely, rather than performing a routine induction. However, some hospitals will provide postdate testing for private patients. In a pilot program at Women's Hospital of Long Beach, California, for example, doctors were encouraged to send their private postdate mothers to the hospital for regular contraction stress tests; among the first 679 deliveries in the pilot program, there was not a single perinatal death. The 25 percent Cesarean rate, while higher than that at Women's Hospital in Los Angeles, was certainly lower than usual in private practice for postdate mothers. Obviously there is still much to be done to reduce Cesarean rates for postmature pregnancies, but in the meantime the contraction stress test is a reliable approach. Discuss this with your doctor.

Make Love, Not Cesareans

Finally, as Nancy Cohen points out in *Silent Knife*, folk wisdom maintains that one unusually reliable way to stimulate the start of labor when babies are overdue is to make love. It is not necessary to have intercourse if that is uncomfortable; what counts it that one way or another, the mother be stimulated to orgasm—preferably several times.

This idea makes perfect physiological sense; if it is now "scientifically recognized" that stimulating the nipples can cause adequate contractions for a test, more stimulation can only cause the mother's body to produce more oxytocin. The only caution would be that since most "postmature" pregnancies are a matter of misdating or of the baby's simply keeping quite healthily to its own schedule, you don't need to start right at your presumed due date, but can wait until the pregnancy is clearly overdue. But if you are facing the imminent threat of induced labor, make love every day. Similarly, doctors at Letterman Army Medical Center in San Francisco recently reported that half of full-term mothers instructed to gently massage their breasts with a warm, moist cloth for one hour three times a day, went into labor within seventy-two hours. You certainly don't need a scientific study to assure you that making love and massage are better than a Cesarean!

"Older" Mothers

In the past decade, a major trend in childbearing has been for women to postpone pregnancy past age thirty. In 1982 in New York City, for example, for the first time in history, more than 25 percent of first-time mothers were over thirty. The course of labor of "older" mothers—variously defined as over age thirty, thirty-five, or forty—has not been well researched. Probably not more than twenty studies in the past twenty years have attempted to define whether "elderly primagravidas" —the tasteless medical term for an older woman having a first birth—are at special risk. (By contrast, the available research on breech deliveries, which constitute only 4 percent of births, would fill a library shelf.)

Despite the dearth of research, obstetricians generally appear to believe that one thing happens to labor as women get older—it becomes unimaginably abnormal, even dangerous. "[Medical] authors have waxed poetic in their descriptions of the obstetric patient, aged forty to forty-five and above," one obstetrician dryly writes. "These premenopausal, truly elderly, geriatric, postmature women in their reproductive senescence are in the twilight of the reproductive period. *William's Obstetrics* [the major obstetrics textbook] states that the frequency of prolonged labor is increased because of uterine dysfunction and apparent cervical rigidity." These presumptions aside, in actual fact older mothers have changed from a group of harassed and tired women in a fifth or sixth pregnancy to career women who have planned a late pregnancy, have taken good care of themselves, and are in excellent health. Birth weight is a prime indication of a normal pregnancy. In the past decade, the percentage of low-birth-weight infants, with all the attendant health problems, has declined more rapidly for first-time mothers over age thirty *than for any other age group.* If you are having your first baby after thirty, you can have an enjoyable pregnancy and natural labor. But look carefully to find a doctor who will treat you like the normal, healthy woman you are.

Physician Biases

In 1964, Dr. Friedman studied the presumed problems of maternal age by analyzing 3,329 first-time older mothers. He noted, first, that doctors had heavily sedated 52.6 percent of mothers over age thirty-five—compared with 30.8 percent of those aged eighteen to thirty-five. And, even though 85 percent of the babies in both groups were normal weight, doctors diagnosed 11.2 percent of older mothers as having fetopelvic disproportion but only 7.8 percent of those eighteen to thirty-five years old. Either pelvises shrink when women reach age thirty-five, Dr. Friedman noted sardonically, or physician "criteria for evaluations changed with age [and] serious biases were being introduced into judgments."

The only real differences in the labor of older mothers which Friedman could document were an 8.3 percent rate of breech babies—it is well recognized that more infants of older mothers do remain in a breech position—and a 4.4 percent rate of detached (abruptio) placenta, an emergency which requires a Cesarean unless the birth is almost complete. Just 1.1 percent of younger mothers developed abruptio placenta. Since the placenta evidently may detach too soon when an anesthetized woman pushes too hard, we may well ask whether overmedication of the older women might have contributed to their problems with abruptio placenta.

Friedman's study found a 20.6 percent Cesarean rate

among the older mothers—very high for that time. He believed that had doctors allowed them to labor as long as younger mothers, their Cesarean rate would have been 7 percent. Also, he found that second-stage labor —after dilation, when the baby is actually being pushed out—tended to be slightly prolonged in older mothers, but that in 90 percent of these cases the mothers had been oversedated. "There was little doubt," he concluded, "that the increased numbers of dysfunctional labor in the older patients was iatrogenic [caused by doctors] in origin."

Most Labor Normally

In a similar vein, Dr. Robert J. Sokol, then at the University of Rochester School of Medicine, found no important differences in birth complications in women aged forty-five and older when compared with younger mothers with the same number of children. The older mothers he studied, however, also had more breech infants. While 75 percent of their abnormal labors occurred with breech deliveries, even with breeches, almost half the abnormal labor patterns started *after* the mothers were given the narcotic meperidine. Younger mothers did not have slowed labor after taking meperidine, but doctors gave them smaller doses. The older mothers, in sum, had quite normal labor except when there was an extenuating circumstance such as a breech baby or oversedation—or, usually, both.

For older mothers who have a child many years after a first one, the new technology of birth—the monitors, sonar, scalp sampling—may be especially frightening. They have, after all, already had a baby without needing any of this. On the other hand, despite the radical change in the birth environment, today's emphasis on knowledge and birth education may come as a pleasant surprise to mothers who also remember the real fear of just plunging into birth without any preparation. One mother, who recently had her second child after a delay of seventeen years, is a good case in point. "The first time," she says, "I had a totally adolescent attitude toward pain. I thought if you were sure of yourself as a woman, you could just eliminate pain. Needless to say, that's totally untrue. Also, I didn't know anything about the physiology of birth. Years ago, you waited for the doctor to give his scholarly lecture about the birth—if he felt like it. Otherwise, no one told you to learn anything. Yes, monitors and technology can intimidate you, but I felt being informed was a good protection and helped me have a better experience. I had heard about the increase in Cesareans, but somehow I felt that at my age, knowing better what I was doing, I just wasn't going to end up with a frivolous Cesarean."

Today's older mother, then, has many advantages that can help her work toward a normal delivery despite physician biases. Most important, she is probably very healthy. She will be well prepared for the birth and have had career or life experiences that have made her well accustomed to dealing with people and analyzing alternatives—abilities that will help her enormously in choosing a doctor and hospital.

Herpes and Birth

Unfortunately, another growing group of mothers in the United States is not so healthy: the millions of women of childbearing age who already have genital herpes or who develop herpes during pregnancy. If you are one of these women you will want to discuss your condition with your doctor and to understand your situation as thoroughly as possible. *Active* herpes virus in the genital area or birth canal at the time of birth can seriously infect babies, causing brain damage, blindness, or death. A Cesarean section is *mandatory* if you have visible lesions at the time of delivery. But the threat to babies has by no means risen in proportion to the herpes epidemic. Active lesions during pregnancy —whether from a new infection or from the flare-up of an old infection—almost never infect infants before birth; in fact, even though upward of 20 million Americans are now said to have contracted herpes, there are still fewer than ten recorded cases in the entire world medical literature of a baby having been infected *before* birth.

Moreover, relatively few women who have herpes need Cesareans. Most herpes episodes are over in a few weeks; in nearly all cases, herpes still active at delivery will advertise itself in sores which can be seen by the doctor or mother. When sores are visible, a Cesarean will be scheduled, usually before the start of labor so that the baby retains the protection of the amniotic sac.* When there are no sores, the mother is a candidate for normal delivery. There is, however, an unfortunate twist known as asymptomatic shedding—when latent herpes continues to shed virus in amounts so small that no lesions form.

Testing for Asymptomatic Shedding

About 4 percent of women who have once had visible herpes may also have shedding episodes during the course of pregnancy. But what does this mean? In the first place, there are no real data on the risk shedding poses to infants—although any risk seems to be minuscule. With herpes rampant among women of child-bearing age, thousands of American women give birth every day to healthy, unaffected babies even though they may be shedding herpes virus. Also, there is no reliable test to determine whether a woman is shedding virus right at term; most shedding episodes are probably quite brief and over within hours. Current tests, depending on the laboratory technique and the concentration of shedding, take from two to five days to confirm the presence of active virus. Obviously, tests taken days ahead can no more tell whether a woman is still shedding at term—or conversely, whether she has started shedding just at term—than yesterday's weather forecast can predict rain for next week.

---

* If there are visible herpes sores and the amniotic sac breaks prematurely, the woman must call her doctor or go to the hospital right away. In this situation, most authorities feel a Cesarean should be performed within four hours to be sure the infection doesn't spread to the baby.

Nonetheless, finding asymptomatic shedders has become almost a sideline in obstetrics. Most women who have herpes will be advised to have weekly tests after about the thirty-fifth week of pregnancy. The test procedure is straightforward—the doctor simply swabs the genital area as he does for a Pap smear—but many observers wonder whether much is gained except to frighten mothers. Some doctors may also use a Pap test for herpes during the delivery. While it gives results in hours, the Pap test is not as sensitive as viral cultures and sometimes suggests active shedding when none exists.

If a woman has shedding episodes during the last weeks of pregnancy, or a "positive" Pap test at the delivery, a Cesarean may be suggested. But obstetricians themselves find the tests ludicrously unreliable, and wonder whether Cesareans are necessary after shedding episodes. Dr. Raymond S. Corwin of Good Samaritan Hospital in Portland, Oregon, has noted that his hospital, like hundreds of others, has not seen a single herpes-infected baby in ten years, yet fears and inconclusive testing caused almost a tenfold increase in Cesareans for herpes mothers between 1979 and 1980 alone. "It appears," he said, "that a child born to a caucasian Seattle woman in her mid-twenties in the middle to upper-middle socioeconomic class has no significant risk of neonatal herpes but that both the infant and its mother have a very definite risk of Cesarean section with its attendant morbidity and mortality."

For the time being, however, it is hard to see what other course doctors can take. "It's pathetic but true," comments an obstetrician involved in herpes research, "that in the current legal climate, most decisions about herpes and pregnancy are based not on medical expediency, but fear of lawsuits." Obviously, each case must be considered individually. If a woman has had a severe primary herpes infection and, since then, has had several recurrences, her doctor's decision both about a Cesarean and about the need for weeks of tests might be different than if she had one mild herpes outbreak years ago and the disease has since been latent.

Does shedding always mean a Cesarean? The obstetrician researching herpes says that, even though his hospital's policy is to recommend Cesareans after shedding episodes in late pregnancy, he would have "no trouble" responding to a request for a vaginal delivery from a mother who had been appropriately counseled—and, also, had signed a release, assuming legal responsibility for her mode of delivery.

Millions Have Normal Births

Millions of mothers who have herpes have also had natural births and healthy babies. As with breech deliveries, however, the question of normal delivery for herpes mothers has become so volatile that doctors do not always act reasonably or in accordance with the medical evidence favoring normal birth. During her first pregnancy, for example, Lesa Williams, a mother who then lived in Kansas, had three outbreaks of lesions from a latent case of herpes. While she did have a negative Pap smear a week before the delivery, her doctor was unwilling to try labor and scheduled a Cesarean even though there was then no evidence of active virus. During her second pregnancy a year and a half later, she did not develop any lesions and her doctor was willing to try labor. But her history of herpes and a previous Cesarean sent the hospital staff into a remarkably unprofessional tailspin. Not only did the head nurse on the obstetrics floor march into the delivery room and yell at Lesa that she was taking a big chance on rupturing her uterus but, afterward, the hospital kept Lesa and her very healthy new baby in "quarantine for herpes"—probably a new concept in medicine considering that neither of them had active virus.

Lesa and the baby were assigned a separate room, which they weren't allowed to leave, and her husband decided to get a cot and spend the night with them. "Every time the nurses came in and out they wore gloves and masks," she says. "When my husband just wanted to go down the hall to the soft drink machine, they wouldn't let him out. It made us feel strange. I do have to say that they stopped that the next morning and apologized and said they had gone overboard."

Despite the hospital's hostility, Lesa Williams recalls this birth as "the most wonderful experience," compared with a Cesarean. "Luckily I had my mother and husband for moral support, and the doctor kept reassuring me," she adds. "It was thirty-eight hours of labor, but I was just really pleased. I felt like I was part of the delivery, and the baby was fine. I remember, afterward, we called my mother-in-law. 'Well,' I said, 'natural is the way to go.' 'If you can say that after thirty-eight hours,' she said, 'you must be right.'"

Help on the Horizon

Part of the solution, obviously, lies with better test procedures—which, fortunately, may be imminent. In February 1983, Genetic Systems, a Seattle firm, announced a new twenty-minute herpes test, and the National Institutes of Health announced a twenty-four-hour test, which they hoped to reduce to a ten-minute procedure within months. As these fast procedures become available, mothers can be reliably tested at the start of delivery, minimizing unneeded Cesareans.

Diabetic Mothers

In the past decade, the dramatic improvement in survival of infants with diabetic mothers has been a real triumph for obstetrics, but one that has also placed an enormous burden on medicine. Mothers must monitor their diet and insulin levels closely to prevent the blood-sugar swings that threaten pregnancy, often causing miscarriage or stillbirth. Often they are hospitalized for months, and to avoid danger at the end of pregnancy, the babies are routinely delivered a week or two early. At many institutions, the primary Cesarean rate for diabetic mothers is 50 percent or more, and the premature infants must be kept in the intensive-care nursery. All told, one baby's birth can cost as much as $40,000. But medical costs aside, the joy for diabetic mothers in having a full-term pregnancy and normal baby is especially compelling. "These mothers want to be like everyone else," emphasizes Dr. Radoslav Jovanovic, a New York obstetrician who works with his wife, Lois, a diabetes specialist. "For them, to have a normal baby and a normal birth is an unbelievable dream. There is endless joy in their expression."

Controlling Blood Sugar

The prerequisite to a normal delivery is a normal pregnancy. If you are diabetic, you will be interested in the work of Dr. Lois Jovanovic, prominent among the leaders of a revolution in health care for diabetic mothers—a revolution which promises to allow most of them to reach term. In her pilot study at New York Hospital in 1981, fifty-two diabetic women were hospitalized for a week in early pregnancy. They were taught to test their own blood glucose (sugar) levels seven times a day and to inject themselves with insulin between three and five times daily (rather than the usual once) at the intervals needed to keep their glucose constantly adjusted. They also received expert nutritional guidance. Although none of the women in the pilot study had graduated from high school, they learned this complex routine readily—Dr. Jovanovic calls diabetic mothers "exquisitely motivated patients" —and kept to it faithfully at home for the rest of the pregnancy. All had healthy babies with no fetal dis-

tress, jaundice, excess weight, or other problems typical of a diabetic pregnancy. In Apgar scores and other
standard measures of infant well-being, the fifty-two
infants of these diabetics were healthier than babies
born to a control population of non-diabetic mothers
who were also clinic patients at New York Hospital!

Five centers (see Appendix for list) throughout the
United States are now experimenting with the same
plan—but now they are training the mothers in home
care even before conception. By starting earlier, mothers avoid the glucose irregularities in early pregnancy
which evidently cause spine and heart deformities in
some children of diabetics. (Babies of diabetics are,
however, not automatically destined to have diabetes;
their risk for diabetes is only somewhat higher than
that for children of non-diabetic mothers and fathers.)
In Dr. Lois Jovanovic's view, it takes about thirty-five
hours of instruction for diabetic mothers to learn to care
for themselves properly at home during pregnancy.
Ideally, she says, they should learn home care and have
normal blood glucose tests for at least two months prior
to trying to conceive.

"It might seem like a lot of trouble, but it really
wasn't hard," says Dale Stillman, a New Jersey mother
who has had two healthy sons while on home treatment. With Dr. Radoslav Jovanovic as her obstetrician,
she also had normal deliveries both times. "It's really
ironic. There I was, a diabetic, injecting myself with
insulin five times a day, and I had a normal delivery,
while, with the general Cesarean rate so high, every
single one of my friends who had a baby recently had
surgery. With Ryan, the labor was a little difficult—

seventeen hours—but with Travis, it was only six hours and I had no drugs at all."

It is clear that most diabetic women can, with proper care, have virtually normal pregnancies. Although the special treatment is not yet routinely available, other hospitals with similar treatment plans have reported success comparable to that at New York Hospital. But, unfortunately, Cesarean rates for diabetic mothers are still very high. A few hospitals have curtailed their "arbitrary early delivery" policies; Yale–New Haven Hospital, for example, has cut its primary Cesarean rate for diabetic mothers to 30 percent. In Europe, the Institute of Obstetrics and Gynecology in Milan, which began treating diabetic women as outpatients several years ago, lets 90 percent of its diabetic mothers go to term and has an 18 percent primary Cesarean rate. But these are exceptions. For the diabetic mothers in Dr. Lois Jovanovic's group, the Cesarean rate was 92 percent, in part because obstetricians at New York Hospital still insisted on delivering most of the babies before term.

"There's been a sort of Catch-22 about it," she observes. "The obstetricians say to me, 'You're giving me so much healthier babies than I used to get with these mothers, why should I take the least chance?' What I say is that normal blood sugars—which is what we are maintaining—make a normal pregnancy. But, you know, medicine is divided into specialties, and people tend to only believe their own. I don't think the obstetricians will be convinced until an obstetricians' group supervises a similar study."

Dr. Radoslav Jovanovic, meanwhile, has worked on taking very sick diabetic mothers—those with kidney deterioration, vascular disease, and other severe complications—to term. In a pilot group, only one of twenty-two mothers was induced before forty weeks and the Cesarean rate was 40 percent. "Next time around, I want to bring down the Cesareans further, but this time I wanted to be sure about mothers in this condition going to term. However, with blood sugar well controlled during pregnancy, all the babies turned out wonderfully, so I'm convinced."

Interestingly, with this group of very sick women, Dr. Jovanovic found that the most helpful method of monitoring fetal status was to teach the mothers to stop several times a day for a few minutes and count fetal movements carefully—a technique known as a "fetal activity test." Although the mothers also had backup non-stress testing using electronic monitors, he concluded the monitors gave him no more useful information than did the mothers' movement counts. Fetal activity testing, Jovanovic believes, while not yet widely employed, perhaps holds a key to the easy, cost-effective methods of fetal surveillance needed not only for diabetic pregnancies but for postmature and other risk pregnancies.

What does this mean for you if you are diabetic? First, try to find a diabetes specialist who really understands home care during pregnancy before you even try to conceive. If you have difficulty obtaining really good diabetic care, perhaps personnel at one of the five major centers now working on home care could recommend a specialist near you. Or, because new treatments are often better known in an academic setting, contact your nearest medical school. With luck, a diabetes specialist there may already be working with an obstetrician who has come to appreciate the potential of home treatment. Realistically, however, if you want a normal birth you may have to push hard for it.

"I think you have to expect the obstetricians to be cautious," comments Donald Coustan, an obstetrician who was instrumental in Yale–New Haven Hospital's home treatment program and is now at Women and Infants Hospital in Providence, Rhode Island. "When you talk about unnecessary Cesareans for this population where early delivery with Cesareans has, in the past, made the difference between life and death for so many, it's not like talking about unnecessary Cesareans in the general population. The obstetricians will want to be very convinced before they massively change over. We still see lots of diabetic mothers in very poor control, and then there's no choice. Also, these mothers are so happy to get live babies, a Cesarean is not as traumatic as it can be for other mothers; it doesn't cause the mourning. Many have already miscarried or thought they would never have children, and they ask for a Cesarean because they're worried about a vaginal birth. I mean, sometimes, when I'm the one who says, 'Come on, let's try it from below,' I feel as though it's the mother who's humoring me."

Clearly, diabetic mothers should have confidence that their prospects for healthy pregnancy and normal delivery have changed dramatically. Most important, however, the good prenatal care which now allows most of them to consider normal delivery is the same care which so enhances the health of their babies even before the birth.

Twins and More

From time to time, the happiness—and the problems —of birth are multiplied by the appearance of more than one baby; twins, which occur in about one in ninety births, are the most common multiple births. Although mothers of twins are increasingly given Cesareans, the condition and position of the babies vary so much that it is clear that automatic Cesareans simply don't solve the problems of twins. For example, Mt. Sinai Hospital in Toronto increased its Cesarean rate for twins from 16 percent to 41 percent between 1975 and 1979—only to see perinatal deaths triple. While perinatal mortality has since decreased and many of the excess deaths occurred among premature twins, the point remains that experience and good training are at least as important as the type of delivery. If you are expecting twins, make sure your doctor is skilled and confident about multiple births. Delivering twins by Cesarean requires skillful manipulation, and unfortunately, it may be that if doctors are not well enough trained and are nervous about vaginal deliveries for these babies, they may not have the confidence to perform Cesareans well either.

The position of the babies will be important to the mode of delivery. Both twins may be head down, both may be breeches, or as frequently happens, there is one in each position. Detailed analysis of twin births over a number of years at the Obstetrical Perinatal Cooperative in Brooklyn has shown no difference in perinatal mortality for first or second twins who are head down, whether they are delivered by Cesarean or vaginally; when delivered vaginally, however, the babies did have better Apgar scores. When either the first or second twin was a breech, there was a slight improvement in survival with Cesarean deliveries, but no improvement in Apgar scores. Mothers should also be aware that when the first twin is head down and the second is breech, experienced doctors can often turn the second fetus even while the mother is in labor, bringing it to a vertex position and improving its survival while avoiding a Cesarean.

If you know that you are expecting triplets—which occur in about one in 8,000 births—or even more babies, seek care from hospitals and doctors well accustomed to managing multiple births. These deliveries demand topnotch skill. The most experienced hospitals do not seem to regard Cesareans as at all mandatory. At the Sloane Hospital for Women in New York City, which has specialized in managing multiple births, half of the thirty-five triplet, quadruplet, and quintuplet births there over a sixteen-year period were Cesareans and half were vaginal deliveries. "The mode of delivery does not seem to play any particular role insofar as outcome is concerned," doctors at Sloane concluded. "In experienced hands, vaginal delivery should be attempted unless there is a medical indication for Cesarean section."

Getting the Support You Need

Clearly, for many mothers routinely branded "high risk," normal birth may be preferable in itself—certainly this is true for most previous Cesarean mothers —or normal birth may be possible because doctors have learned to treat difficult pregnancies as normally as possible. The turned breech baby, the well-controlled diabetic mother, and the properly managed postmature mother are all examples of pregnancies where a hospital's or doctor's success at normal birth reflects marked success at promoting healthy pregnancies and infant survival.

Feeling Overwhelmed

Still, if you are embarking on a "new" course for a difficult pregnancy, you may feel somewhat alone and overwhelmed. It would be nice, of course, if you could fully depend on family and friends for emotional support, but this is not always possible. Your own mother may have been raised with the firm belief that "it's not nice to question the doctor," and by now so many sisters-in-law and cousins have had Cesareans that they may feel embarrassed or threatened when a woman close to them questions the need for a Cesarean birth.

Many women are especially vulnerable during pregnancy. Rather than trying to get support from the unconverted, seek out friends or organizations who already have a good understanding of normal birth. Look for local childbirth support groups, or ask your obstetrician if he or she can introduce you to a woman with your own problem—whether it be diabetes, herpes, a previous Cesarean, or a breech—who has recently had a normal birth. There is no greater encouragement than talking to a woman who already has a healthy baby and can describe exactly what to expect during the delivery.

Study, Learn, and Stay Calm

You may also feel discouraged because many doctors are so far behind in the advances being made in normal births for high-risk mothers, but try to remember that it is very difficult for doctors to change the procedures which they were taught, even if their methods are now outdated. If, after polite but clear conversations, the doctor unmistakably opposes your expectations, it is simply time to look elsewhere. Don't waste energy on arguments. Even leaders of the childbirth education movement say that during pregnancy they felt so vulnerable it was hard for them to confront a doctor. Mothers should not be afraid to be even a little cowardly to get what they want—namely to keep calm and have a normal birth. Ask your husband or friends to run interference for you if necessary, as Anne Squadron did when changing doctors in the last month of pregnancy.

If you are a high-risk mother, you will have to work hard to be well informed. With the terrific advances being made in the care of diabetics, mothers with herpes, and postmature pregnancies, you should be able to find plenty of reading material at a medical library. Go over recent journals for the latest information about your situation. But finally, no matter how well informed you are, and no matter how excellent and helpful the medical professionals you find, there will almost inevitably be times when there are no clear-cut answers to your questions and you will be afraid of making any decision in case it's the wrong one. Swings between fears and high hopes are natural for "risk" mothers. Try to be calm, and simply do what feels right. Pat Nolan, a rehabilitation supervisor at a psychiatric hospital who had her first baby in October 1982, found herself in just such a situation. Although she and her husband, Mark Slifer, were planning for their baby to be delivered at Albert Einstein Hospital in New York City, they took Lamaze classes locally in the town of Carmel where they lived. When they learned the baby was a breech, the first person they thought to question closely was the Lamaze instructor.

"We asked her what it meant for the delivery, but she refused to discuss it at all," Mark comments. "We later learned that the local hospital, where she's a nurse, had a policy of Cesareans for all breeches, so I guess it was a conflict for her and she didn't know what to say. But that really made us crazy. We thought it was simple and we began to realize we had a big problem."

"Our doctor, who happened to be in group practice with Dr. Schulman, tried to turn the baby and couldn't," Pat says. "Then she called in Dr. Schulman and he couldn't turn it either, so they told me they would try a vaginal delivery, but I should also go to a class about Cesareans so I could learn about the operation. Well, I went to the class and I saw the film and I came out crying. However, I finally pulled myself out of that, and then I went out and got a whole new batch of books about birth—this time about Cesareans. Now I didn't know any longer. If I tried a vaginal delivery, which I really wanted, was I doing the right thing for the baby?"

Pat's doctor agreed to let her try a vaginal delivery. Her labor lasted twenty hours; for the last two hours the hospital had an operating room on standby for surgery. "Looking back, what you can see is it could have gone either way," Mark recalls. "We wouldn't have been upset if there was a Cesarean by then, because the hospital tried so hard. By that, I don't mean just the doctors. The nurses, too. Everybody. They just went out of their way."

Finally, the baby was born naturally.

"I would say I was still in conflict about trying a vaginal right until my labor began," Pat acknowledges. "But when I got into it, it was really worth it. I had such a sense of accomplishment. I was up and walking two hours after it was over and just look what I got."

A healthy, alert baby boy named Sean.

Chapter Four

CESAREAN RISKS

""There is no question," Dr. Emanuel Friedman wrote in the Harvard Medical School's *Medical Forum* in June 1981, "that a completely normal vaginal delivery is to be preferred because it presents negligible perils to mother and baby. By contrast, a Cesarean section is major surgery. Whereas the risks associated with Cesarean operations today are small compared to what they were years ago, they are still ever-present and cannot be ignored."

If a problem arises in your pregnancy, you will want to have as clear an understanding as possible of Cesarean risks—as well as of the times when there is good evidence that the benefits to your baby and yourself may outweigh the risks of surgical delivery. To spend a lot of time questioning doctors and studying alternatives may seem like a lot of trouble. It is important to remember why you are making this effort—to find the best medical care and make the best choices for your child's birth.

It may seem a daunting prospect to find the right balance between the risks and potential benefits of Cesarean surgery, because two patients have to be considered; what is better for the mother may not always be best for the infant or vice versa. On the whole, however, the evidence clearly favors normal labor for the great majority of deliveries; and, most important, there are very few instances where either the mother or baby is so ill that a Cesarean should be scheduled before the mother has even tried a normal delivery. In other words, most mothers can insist on at least having a genuine, ungrudging chance at labor.

Let's look more closely at what is known—and what is not known—about the risks and the benefits of Cesarean surgery.

Risks to Mothers

While it is reassuring that fewer than four hundred mothers a year die in childbirth in the United States, it is *not* reassuring to know that the death rate for Cesarean mothers is two to four times higher than for vaginal births. Research both in the United States and Europe has confirmed again and again that at least half of maternal deaths during Cesarean section are caused by the operation itself—and are not simply the result of the mother's being in poor health. A review panel of obstetricians in Georgia recently found that, of sixteen maternal deaths during Cesarean section, nine resulted directly from the operation, rather than from the mother's condition. Moreover, some authorities believe that, because the mode of delivery is not always stated on maternal death certificates, the true rate of maternal deaths during Cesarean section is at least twenty times higher than commonly thought.

Anesthesia

The majority of maternal deaths during Cesarean section follow from the complications of using general anesthesia. Cesareans are actually one of the few operations where doctors have several choices of anesthesia. Cesareans may be performed under general— or inhalation—anesthesia, under "regional" anesthesia, and under an impressively safe but little-used method of local anesthesia. Although local anesthesia seems almost incapable of killing the mother or child, unfortunately probably not a dozen obstetricians in the United States use it regularly.

Between the generals and regionals which are currently the standard choices, regionals are obviously safer. Inhalation anesthesia may cause the mother to regurgitate gastric acid from her stomach and breathe it into her lungs; by contrast, fatal aspiration of the stomach contents is extremely rare during regional anesthesia. Except when general anesthesia is medically indicated—it is faster in an emergency and is better for mothers with some medical conditions, particularly low blood pressure—regionals are usually preferred. Also, with regional anesthesia, mothers are awake and can watch the birth. However, the initial problem of needle placement—the anesthesia must be carefully directed to the base of the spinal cord—and getting a regional to "take" is trickier than rendering a woman unconscious with inhaled gas. One of the disturbing aspects of the Cesarean explosion is that it has so outpaced the personnel trained to administer regionals that more and more generals have had to be used. At major teaching hospitals surveyed between 1970 and 1975, the number of Cesareans performed with generals went up from 32 percent to 45 percent.

At present, training seems to be catching up and the preponderance of generals is subsiding. Still, there are areas of the country where, as one anesthesiologist puts it, "you couldn't get a regional for a million dollars."

What you are even more unlikely to get is local anesthesia. With this technique, the mother is simply given several shots of a painkiller—usually the Novocain familiar to everyone from dentist visits—in the abdomen. Because she can still move and breathe so easily, and because the dosage is so low, this method is extremely safe for both her and the baby. It is also relatively easy to administer. However, while acknowledging the superior safety of local anesthesia, doctors routinely write in the medical journals that they doubt they could get their patients to accept it. Yet Dr. Ranney, for one, has used local anesthesia for most of his Cesarean deliveries for thirty years. He has quite a different view of both the intelligence and motivation of mothers. "I've never known a single woman to refuse a few needle pricks when she knew it was better for both her baby and herself," he comments.

Infection

If anesthesia complications are the most dangerous for Cesarean mothers, infections are the most common complication of surgery. Even with the prophylactic use of antibiotics—that is, giving antibiotics at the time of surgery, rather than waiting to see if the mother develops an infection—about 20 to 40 percent of first-time Cesarean mothers will have such problems. But only 1 to 2 percent of mothers with vaginal deliveries develop infections. Not only is this a striking difference in itself, but many doctors wonder what will happen if the continuing high Cesarean rate causes the use of antibiotics to reach a scale that encourages antibiotic-resistant strains of bacteria to evolve. As a result, concerned doctors will not give preventive antibiotics to all Cesarean mothers—only to those who they suspect will be at risk for infection. "I mean, we've got the drugs now," Dr. Haverkamp of Denver General notes, "but who knows when the bugs will outwit them if we keep using them this way?"

Endometritis, an infection of the lining of the uterus, is the most common infection, followed by urinary-tract and wound infections, pneumonia and other respiratory diseases. (The respiratory infections are another effect of general anesthesia.) Although about 80 percent of the operative site infections respond to antibiotics in a relatively short time, it is by no means unusual for mothers to be rehospitalized to have wounds cleaned and resutured, or even for various in-

ternal infections to become very serious; in the Los
Angeles Women's Hospital random study, two of the
148 breech-Cesarean mothers had to have hysterectomies because of severe infection even though they had
been given prophylactic antibiotics.

Hemorrhage

About 10 percent of Cesarean mothers hemorrhage
so much that they require a transfusion. Most of the
hemorrhaging is the unavoidable consequence of surgery, but, because the lower abdomen is densely
packed with organs and blood vessels, surgical accidents in that area can result in severe bleeding.

In the Women's Hospital study, fourteen of the 148
Cesarean mothers needed transfusions—twelve of
them two or more times—compared with one transfusion for the sixty vaginally delivered mothers. Although no Cesarean mother in that study required a
hysterectomy because of hemorrhaging, hysterectomy
is in fact occasionally necessary, depending on both the
site of the bleeding and whether it was caused by surgical error.

Other complications of Cesarean surgery—bladder
and intestinal punctures, intestinal obstruction, and
various persistent infections—have almost certainly
been underestimated. Most studies only look at the
condition of Cesarean mothers while they remain at
the hospital, and have not focused on later readmis-
sions and treatment for those who were actually the
sickest.

Emotional Consequences

As undeniable and persistent as are the physical consequences of Cesarean section, it may be that the subtle emotional consequences of this surgery affect mothers more deeply over the long term. What is the effect of a childbirth fraught with physical pain, anxiety, the shock of surgery, and separation of the mother and new baby immediately after the delivery? Dr. Dugald Baird, the obstetrician in Aberdeen, Scotland, was perhaps the first person to seriously consider this question. When, in 1955, he recommended modestly increasing the local 1.1 percent primary Cesarean rate, he wanted to be sure not to unknowingly recommend a course that would disturb women's attitudes toward children and childbirth. For four years, he followed a large group of first-time mothers: those who had had easy vaginal deliveries within twelve hours of labor, those who had difficult forceps deliveries after long labor, and those with Cesareans. Nearly all the vaginally delivered mothers, whether their labor was easy or excruciating, went on to have a second child; but three-quarters of the Cesarean mothers stopped having children. "Cesarean section," Dr. Baird concluded, "appears to have a deterrent effect which is not found after any form of vaginal delivery."

Since then, there have been many attempts to try to clarify the emotional risks of Cesarean section—how serious they may be and how long-lasting. Yet emotional causes and effects are so difficult to define, it is difficult to arrive at definite conclusions. "The problem is that you're constantly dealing with different situations," comments Dr. Muriel Sugarman, an infant and child psychiatrist at the Harvard Medical School and Beth Israel Hospital in Boston. "The reaction may be very different when a mother truly knows a Cesarean saved her child than when she has good reason to think 'some jerk botched it.' A colleague and I were discussing using animal experiments to try to get some consistent observations but she said, 'You know, if we treat animal mothers during birth the way we treat human mothers, they'll just reject or outrightly kill their young.' " And, in fact, the outcome of what appears to be the only Cesarean experiment done on monkeys is highly disturbing. In this experiment, seven laboratory-reared rhesus monkeys were given Cesareans. Although laboratory-reared female monkeys do not have as strong a maternal instinct as wild monkeys, they will usually accept their vaginally delivered infants; but not one of the seven mothers—even those who had already successfully raised a vaginally born baby—would care for or even touch its Cesarean-born infant.

Meanwhile, research with human mothers has suggested that, leaving aside questions of the pain and shock of surgery, unnecessary separation of mother and newborn may sometimes impair a mother's "normal" reaction to her baby. This research centers on the fascinating process of mother-infant bonding and the groundbreaking work of Marshall Klaus and John Kennell, then professors of pediatrics at the Case Western Reserve University Medical School.

Bonding

Bonding between mother and child occurs in the first few days, and especially in the first hour, after birth. During those first hours, infants and mothers will follow each other in what Klaus and Kennell have dubbed a kind of "primeval dance" of mutual gazing and touching motions. The behavior appears instinctive, or programmed into us as a way for mothers and infants to introduce themselves and become attached.

In their early research, Klaus and Kennell allowed one group of new mothers to keep their babies with them for longer periods during the first three days of life than hospital regulations ordinarily allowed. During routine checkups a month later, these mothers handled their infants differently than women whose early contact was limited to the infants' feeding periods. They had significantly more eye-to-eye contact with their babies and fondled them more, and they were also more reluctant to leave their babies. In the interval since Klaus and Kennell conducted their study, we have seen a deluge of research into mother–infant attachment. The results, while not entirely consistent, have led the majority of American hospitals to change their regulations and permit mothers and babies to stay together right after birth; however, the increased Cesarean rate has obviously challenged our new appreciation of bonding.

"With Cesarean birth," Dr. Sugarman has written, "there are the additional problems of post-surgical

pain, healing and fatigue to complicate matters and in
most hospitals the Cesarean mother must also be separated from her infant for twenty-four hours while the
infant is observed for complications. We cannot predict
with certainty which mother-infant pairs will suffer
permanent distortion or diminution of attachment, or
how that can be measured, or what long-range effects
on personality development will result. It behooves us,
then, to treat mother and infant with the care and respect their vulnerability and immense importance de-
serve."

If we cannot measure the extent to which Cesareans
interfere with mother–infant bonding, and even if we
can cite endless examples of parents and children who
overcome bonding disruptions—as witness the love
between adoptive parents and their infants—we also
have endless testimony from Cesarean mothers themselves who feel there was something "wrong" about
their reactions to the birth and to their child. Indeed, it
is because of those emotional reactions—their anger,
their sense of estrangement from the child—that Cesarean mothers across the country have formed
hundreds of mutual-support groups where they can
talk out their feelings.

One important lesson mothers learn from these support groups is that it may take time for even a "well-
adjusted, middle-class" mother to understand her own
reactions to the operation. These are the mothers who
may tell themselves not to complain, just to be thankful
their babies are healthy. Later, however, many of them
realize that emotions are not always so easy to control.
Esther Zorn, the Cesarean Prevention Movement

leader, did not fully understand her own reactions to her Cesarean until her son was a toddler. "Because the birth was so frightening and out of control, I developed an almost obsessive need to control Fred's activities," she recalls, "and I can tell you that we spent some ridiculously unhappy times as he got older. Finally, I came to realize what I was doing and why and got it straightened out. I never had that with my second child, who was a vaginal birth. I am absolutely convinced it was a matter of birth method—not birth order. I could hardly exaggerate the difference. I was always so preoccupied with Fred that if everything wasn't just right, it would set my teeth on edge. I've simply never had that feeling with the second." The combined physical and emotional risks of Cesarean section are major, unrelenting considerations for mothers. "We know enough to know that Cesareans can be deeply disturbing," comments Beth Shearer of C-Sec, Inc., the Massachusetts-based Cesarean support group, "and it's enough to know that. We don't have to have the exact percentage of very upset mothers for that knowledge to be important."

Risks to Babies

In return for the clear risks to mothers, the major payoff of Cesareans is supposed to be better infant survival. Is this the case? While individual Cesareans are certainly sometimes life-saving, there is no reason to think that the Cesarean explosion has improved overall infant survival.

We have already looked at several hospitals where excellent infant survival and low Cesarean rates go hand in hand. These included National Maternity in Dublin, which has kept to a 4.6 percent Cesarean rate, yet deaths for the eight thousand babies a year born there have tumbled almost twice as fast as infant deaths in the United States; or Denver General, which has reduced its Cesarean rate impressively even while enhancing infant survival. Nonetheless, you will often read the claim that, since overall infant survival has improved during the years of the Cesarean explosion, Cesareans must be helping more infants to survive.

Before you accept such a claim about Cesareans, remember that other important factors in maternal and infant care have also changed during the decades of the Cesarean explosion. Probably the most important contemporary factor in improving infant survival is that contraceptives have become widely accepted, thereby encouraging mothers to plan and space children, and making their pregnancies much healthier. Intensive-care nurseries have also enhanced infant survival. But there is little evidence that Cesareans per se are a factor. In fact, a major long-term analysis at Kings County Hospital and Downstate Medical Center in Brooklyn shows just the opposite: infant survival actually improved most during the years Cesarean rates were *lowest*.

Since this is a classic American study of Cesareans and survival, let's examine it more closely. Between them, the two affiliated hospitals—one public and one private—deliver some six thousand babies a year and serve a broad population of both healthy and unhealthy mothers. From 1961 to 1967, when their average Cesarean rate was 6 percent, perinatal mortality dropped consistently every year; but between 1973 and 1977, as the Cesarean rate climbed from 12 percent to 17 percent of births, perinatal mortality at the two hospitals stayed exactly the same. In the face of these figures, any argument about Cesareans and an "overall" contribution to infant survival collapses.

Respiratory Distress

Perhaps one reason the Cesarean increase has not demonstrably improved infant survival is that the tripled Cesarean rate has exposed hundreds of thousands more babies a year to extra risks. Infant deaths attributable to mode of delivery alone—that is, purely to a choice between a vaginal and a Cesarean delivery—are very infrequent; but when 600,000 babies a year are exposed to even a small risk of fetal complications, deaths almost certainly will mount.

The most common avoidable cause of death for infants delivered by Cesarean is respiratory distress, or breathing difficulties. Intensive-care nurseries around the country continue to report that between 3 and 15 percent of their admissions are babies who developed respiratory distress following a Cesarean section. For the most part, these babies simply have immature lungs and were delivered—especially if they were automatic repeat Cesareans—before the start of labor. But more puzzling is that babies with mature lungs still develop respiratory distress. It would seem that the Cesarean operation itself is sometimes the cause of respiratory disease.

Lung Testing

Many obstetricians had assumed that "sophisticated" tests for fetal lung maturity could eliminate respiratory distress as a risk factor for Cesarean infants. Since this has not proven to be the case—testing has lowered the incidence of respiratory distress, but probably will never prevent all cases—the whole subject of respiratory disease is undergoing intense reevaluation.

The major test for fetal lung maturity is the L/S ratio, or ratio of lecithin and sphinogymelin in the lungs. These two chemicals are surfactants which help transport oxygen. However, the test is not easy to do. To obtain the L/S ratio, doctors must insert a long needle, usually with ultrasound as a guide, into the mother's abdomen and remove amniotic fluid for analysis. Not only is this procedure, known as amniocentesis, costly and uncomfortable, but its side effects, although rare, can be serious and include needle punctures of the baby. Not surprisingly, many doctors are reluctant to take L/S ratios routinely for the many mothers—including repeat Cesarean mothers, mothers with herpes lesions, and diabetic mothers—whose Cesareans are scheduled before labor starts. After "several traumatic fetal injuries" from taking L/S ratios, Women's Hospital in New York City has decided, instead, to rely on ultrasound and old-fashioned clinical judgment for assessing fetal age before initiating Cesareans.

If some doctors have stayed away from L/S tests because they think the procedure is problematic, many others still give no thought whatsoever to the prevention of respiratory distress. You may recall, for example, that the Hershey Medical Center in Pennsylvania reported on several babies sent to its intensive-care unit for severe respiratory distress following a Cesarean. In *no* case had the delivering doctor made any special effort—whether ultrasound, consultation, or an L/S test —to determine the true gestational age of the child before scheduling surgery. "These observations are awesome," doctors at Hershey Medical Center concluded, "when one considers the amount of time and effort that must be expended in the management of this condition in neonatal units, the potentially devastating (sometimes fatal) short- and long-term effects on the lives of these infants and their families, and the enormous monetary involvement."

Some doctors also believe there has been a fundamental misunderstanding and that respiratory distress sometimes occurs simply because the baby, no matter how mature, is delivered by Cesarean section. Dr. Richard L. Schreiner, an Indiana pediatrician, was rather startled when, reviewing the records of a local intensive-care nursery, he discovered that 30 percent of the infants admitted for respiratory distress had been judged mature by both an obstetrician and a pediatrician and that several had confirming ultrasound and L/S tests. He has proposed that these babies did not have classical respiratory distress, with direct injury to lung tissue, but a condition known as persistent fetal circulation. "What we *think* happens—no one really knows—is that the blood flow from the right ventricle of the heart to the pulmonary [lung] arteries is inadequate," he says. "The babies will be very sick for five to ten days, sometimes three weeks, and then, usually, they get better for reasons we also don't understand. I wouldn't want to exaggerate the incidence. Estimating conservatively, the 47 babies in the study, transferred from several hospitals, probably came from a pool of about 125,000 births. However, for every sick baby transferred, there would be more not so severely ill. Some people suggest all respiratory distress is preventable by L/S tests. I don't believe that." Mature L/S tests or no, those babies spent up to 156 days in the intensive-care unit. Eighteen had to be put on respirators. One died, and eighteen required further hospitalization after leaving intensive care.

Well over a decade into the Cesarean explosion, respiratory distress is still not well understood; what we do know is that many more Cesarean babies, both mature and immature, die from this disease than vaginally delivered infants—and that every increase in the Cesarean rate therefore puts more babies at risk.

Suspected Deaths from Anesthesia

The question of anesthesia deaths has barely begun to be explored. General anesthesia, which is the most dangerous for mothers, is also the most dangerous for infants. Obstetricians, obstetric nurses, and midwives say they suspect Cesarean infants are occasionally lost to general anesthesia; but we do not have large studies comparing perinatal deaths according to type of anesthesia and the reason for the Cesarean. Probably the best insight we can obtain into infant deaths from anesthesia is to examine Dr. Ranney's lifetime records.

Dr. Ranney's own opinion of anesthesia began with a Cesarean death. "When I first got to Yankton," he recalls, "there was no one specially trained to do obstetric anesthesia. Careful as we were, I thought we were losing infants anyway. In 1951, I had a term normal-weight baby die of respiratory distress after a Cesarean—which I thought was related to general anesthesia—and the next year I lost a term infant with a spinal. The truth is, there is no general anesthesia you can give which doesn't affect the baby immediately, and, with spinals, the physiologic variations among women are so great that the safe dose also varies and you never really know. So, with all these problems, I thought it wise to develop a method of anesthesia I could really control and that wouldn't affect the baby."

The method Dr. Ranney turned to was local anesthesia, giving the mother several—usually twelve— shots of Novocain in the abdomen. Over a period of twenty-five years, 26 percent of babies he delivered by emergency Cesarean died when general anesthesia was used, but only 6 percent died with local anesthesia. While this is not a "scientifically controlled" study—that would require matching mothers closely for age, number of children, and other characteristics, and matching babies for weight, the nature of the emergency, and so on—the mothers were reasonably similar, having Cesareans for pretty much the same reasons, and they were delivered by the same doctor. The message seems clear and not a little chilling; Dr. Ranney believes he could have halved perinatal mortality for emergency Cesarean babies by using local anesthesia for all their births.

This is a crucial issue for Cesarean births in general. Although most Cesarean babies can withstand anesthesia better than the very sick or premature infants typical of emergency deliveries, obviously the increased Cesarean rate—plus the increased use of general anesthesia which has accompanied it—has meant exposing millions of infants to potentially lethal drugs. In reviewing all the Cesareans he has done, Dr. Ranney further noted that almost all babies born under local anesthesia breathed spontaneously, but 97 percent of those delivered under general anesthesia and 64 percent of those delivered under a spinal could not breathe on their own and had to be resuscitated with oxygen, or further measures. In the course of thirty years, Dr. Ranney lost only two mature Cesarean babies, one delivered under a spinal and the other under a general. He has never lost a mature Cesarean baby delivered with a local anesthetic.

"I read all the time in the journals about how this technique with spinals is safe or that agent for inhalation is safe," Dr. Ranney adds, "and maybe that's true in the hands of people writing up articles for medical journals. But, you know, out in the field, you aren't always dealing with the greatest geniuses. You have to take that into account in considering anesthesia effects."

The available facts, while not complete, certainly suggest why it is worth the time for parents to find a good hospital with a low Cesarean rate. If the Cesarean explosion is not causing excess infant deaths, why do so many hospitals which perform relatively few Cesareans have excellent infant survival? Why, in a 1979 study, did the six municipal hospitals in New York City with the highest Cesarean rates have on average 50 percent more perinatal deaths than the six with the lowest Cesarean rates—even though their patient populations were virtually identical in terms of risk factors? Or, how could Dublin Maternity Hospital make such striking gains in infant survival while holding its Cesarean rate to 4.6 percent? As a parent, your own response to these questions is to be certain that your doctor and hospital appreciate Cesarean risks and will not recommend unjustified surgery.

The Best-Justified Cesareans

Emergencies do sometimes occur which justify surgery. We looked at some of these situations briefly in Chapter 1. However, in the rare event that your labor runs into severe trouble, you will want to know more about the circumstances in which a Cesarean is indicated so that you can feel reassured you are accepting the best course for your baby.

Major birth emergencies include prolapse of the umbilical cord, in which the cord enters the birth canal before the infant; placenta previa, in which the placenta is attached to the lower rather than upper uterus; and abruptio placentae, in which the placenta has detached from the wall of the uterus, cutting off the fetus's oxygen supply. Very hard pushing by an overanesthetized mother may contribute to detached placenta; however, the single best-documented cause of both placenta previa and abruptio placentae is maternal smoking; *women who smoke more than a pack of cigarettes a day during pregnancy double their prospects for serious placental complications.*

Although these conditions usually require a Cesarean, the doctor may also be correct in having the mother proceed with a normal birth. For instance, though Cesareans halve infant deaths for cord prolapse, the speed of delivery is also crucial, and the doctor might advise that a mother nearing the end of vaginal birth continue. Placenta previa can be complete, which requires a Cesarean, or partial, which suggests alternatives. In a celebrated recent case in Jackson, Michigan, a hospital obtained a court order directing an "uncooperative" mother with partial placenta previa to appear for treatment—presumably a Cesarean. The woman went to another hospital and had a normal delivery of a healthy nine-pound boy. On the whole, however, such emergencies are not the time to argue. Luckily, they happen rarely.

Cesarean delivery is also frequently advocated for all very premature infants—say, those aged twenty-five to thirty weeks. The condition of these babies after birth is, in fact, an emergency, but there is some doubt whether the available evidence suggests a preferred delivery method for all such infants. Doctors at Yale–New Haven Hospital, in looking at very premature breeches, have reported that vaginal delivery becomes highly problematic only when the baby weighs less than 1,500 grams (3.4 pounds), in part because the mother's cervix simply is not ready for delivery. On the other hand, at McMaster University Medical Centre in Ontario, for breech babies weighing less than 1,000 grams, mortality decreased only 20 percent during a period when their Cesarean rate zoomed from 13 to 50 percent; however, during the same period, mortality for very small vertex babies decreased by 50 percent even though the Cesarean rate for them increased only modestly. To doctors there, these figures hardly argued for the superiority of Cesarean section. "The prematurity itself," they concluded, "with all its accompanying pathophysiology, is so overwhelming that maneuvers involving method of delivery do not alter outcome."

If the amniotic waters are stained green and brown, this means that meconium, a waste substance from the fetal intestines, has been released, and the fetus must be carefully watched for a slowed heartbeat, which could indicate it has inhaled the meconium. Distress related to meconium inhalation may require a Cesarean. Various other abnormal labor and fetal conditions, including dystocia and unexplained distress, have already been discussed. Cesareans may occasionally be warranted in these situations, but in the absence of a clear emergency it obviously becomes harder to justify surgery or even suggest how often it might be crucial. Mothers should remember that, in the absence of emergency, there is usually plenty of time for them to ask questions and try natural measures to put the birth back on track.

Finally, there are the maternal illnesses—prominently diabetes and hypertension—which often justify Cesareans. Although many women with these diseases do deliver normally, when diabetes or hypertension is severe, above-average Cesarean rates clearly contribute to infant survival.

Morbidity

For the most part, research about risks to infants from the mode of delivery has focused on infant mortality. However, we must also be concerned about infant morbidity, or birth-related illnesses or injuries which are not life-threatening. For instance, for every Cesarean baby who died of respiratory distress at the Pennsylvania and Indiana regional intensive-care nurseries, another twenty to forty were severely ill, and there were many more with mild respiratory disease who were never transferred to the central unit. But on the subject of morbidity, the gaps in research are enormous and doctors must make thousands of Cesarean decisions without the basic facts they need.

Brain Damage and Oxygen Deprivation

Worries about brain damage to the infant create great pressure to perform Cesareans. To have a normal child's mental potential impaired through a birth accident is, of course, devastating. Doctors must certainly be concerned about oxygen deprivation which could lead to brain damage; however, fetal monitors have caused considerable confusion between an electronic reading of "distress" and real oxygen deprivation, and many doctors now tend to rush into Cesareans when monitor patterns become slightly irregular.

Unnecessary "distress" Cesareans are probably the most devastating kind. A mother may never be certain whether she had true disproportion or whether her "dysfunctional" labor would have functioned fine if she had been given more time. But a good-to-excellent Apgar score when the baby is born—which is the case in the majority of distress Cesareans—will reveal that the baby was not in imminent danger of brain damage. Not only will both mother and infant have been exposed to the risks of unnecessary surgery, but ironically, considering that the operation was performed to "prevent" brain damage, if general anesthesia was used, the baby will also have been exposed to a drug widely suspected to itself threaten the delicate fetal nervous system.

Unfortunately, there has not been a single study which has followed vaginal and Cesarean children with stressful monitor patterns to school age to evaluate whether either mode of delivery may affect their behavior or intellectual development and motor skills.

But it is worth looking more closely at what evidence we do have about brain damage at birth. Researchers have done a number of experiments with monkeys to try to duplicate difficult vaginal births; interestingly, although monkey fetuses asphyxiated—that is, severely deprived of oxygen—during birth often die, the infants who survive almost invariably have normal brains. These monkey experiments mirror observations of human babies deprived of oxygen by cord or placental accidents. Even when placental ruptures are so severe that the mother goes into shock and the baby's life is at stake, follow-up has shown no unusual IQ or motor deficits among such children by the time they reach school age. While these results obviously do not argue for vaginal birth—a high Cesarean rate does save infant lives here—they do suggest the recuperative powers of the infant brain against oxygen deprivation at the time of delivery.

But most Cesareans performed because the fetal brain is presumably at stake are done not because of cord prolapse or placental rupture, but to guard against potential brain damage when fetal monitors show ambiguous "distress" readings. At this point in obstetrics, no one has the least notion how often or under what conditions distress actually causes brain damage, and there is virtually no way to justify current Cesarean rates by the specter of stress-related brain damage. You will recall the excellent study of distress Cesareans at Denver General Hospital that involved 690 high-risk mothers divided into three groups: some monitored electronically during the delivery, some monitored electronically with fetal scalp sampling as a backup, and the rest monitored by nurses with a stethoscope. The electronically monitored group without scalp sampling had an 18 percent Cesarean rate, and two-thirds of these operations were performed for presumed fetal distress; the group monitored by stethoscope had a 6 percent Cesarean rate, with but a single operation for fetal distress. Yet, average Apgar scores were the same for all the groups of babies. Also, analysis of umbilical-cord blood gases for relative oxygen deprivation again showed no differences between the three groups. In other words, many of the babies in the high Cesarean group had not been deprived of oxygen.

At the University of California at Davis, doctors have made one of the few attempts to follow babies diagnosed as "distressed" on the basis of monitor readings to an age when neurological abnormalities are more easily diagnosed. Of seventy-five babies declared "distressed" according to monitor readings during birth, Apgar scores showed that, whether delivered vaginally or by Cesarean, only seventeen were actually distressed when born. Also, among all seventy-five "distressed" babies, Apgar scores improved slightly with vaginal delivery. The babies were followed for a month or more, and ultimately six were diagnosed as having neurological abnormalities (ranging from cerebral palsy to poor motor skills). Three of these infants were delivered by Cesarean and three vaginally.

Two points of interest about the babies with neurological abnormalities emerged. Although the popular theory is that quick removal of the distressed infant is what prevents neurological abnormalities and justifies Cesareans, five out of six of the abnormal babies were delivered *more quickly* than the average delivery time of distressed babies who turned out to be normal. And, except for a single infant who, a year later, developed unexplained seizures, all the neurologically abnormal babies had been suspected of being in trouble well before the delivery. Either their mothers had been ill or they had displayed weak fetal movements. "Evidence of asphyxia [during birth] was not followed by a neurologic abnormality in the infant unless there was a pre-existing chronic fetal distress," the doctors at Davis concluded.

Generally, then, Cesareans do not seem to protect the neurological development of even the sickest babies. While there is no doubt that oxygen deprivation can be very dangerous, true deprivation and "distress" as now routinely defined in obstetrics are entirely different matters. More likely, doctors who overreact to signs of distress by performing Cesareans immediately do more harm than good.

Brain Damage and Anesthesia

Because the brain, at birth, is one of the least complete organs of the body, there is concern that anesthesia and drugs can interfere with "details" of its final development. All agents commonly used for analgesia and anesthesia during childbirth cross the placenta and reach the baby's brain; because every increase in the Cesarean rate means a direct increase in the use of major anesthesia—and, especially, general anesthesia, which is known to be the most toxic to the nervous system—the question of Cesareans and brain damage is important.

A preliminary analysis of the 400 healthiest Cesarean infants from the Collaborative Perinatal Project, a government study of some 50,000 pregnancies and the later health of the children, showed that 3 percent more of the infants exposed to general anesthesia during the delivery were "neurologically abnormal" at age one than those exposed to regional anesthesia. One study cannot be conclusive—this does seem to be the only attempt to evaluate possible long-term anesthesia effects in a well-controlled study of Cesarean babies— but the idea that general anesthesia is dangerous to brain development receives support from other research.

Because the Collaborative Prenatal Project was started in the late 1950s, inhalation anesthesia was still common for vaginal deliveries. Testing of the 3,500 healthiest vaginally delivered babies at age four months, eight months, and one year suggested that, of all anesthetics and drugs used during childbirth, the inhalation agent, nitrous oxide, had the greatest impact on children. Babies exposed to it were slower to sit, stand, and move around; they tended to be somewhat more irritable and more easily frustrated than other youngsters. Babies born under general anesthesia also tended to have higher blood pressure at one year of age. Nitrous oxide is still used routinely for Cesarean deliveries.

Even more interesting, perhaps, are Dr. Ranney's records. He may be the only doctor in the United States who has tried to review the current health of every Cesarean baby he ever delivered. So far, he has evaluated 232 youngsters, now between one and twenty-four years old. The babies delivered under general anesthesia were twice as likely to later have neurological or behavior abnormalities, such as poor motor skills, gen-

eral slowness in school, and reading and speech difficulties, as those delivered with local anesthesia. Again,
his is not a strict scientific study—in which the children would have to be closely matched according to
the reason for the Cesarean and other factors—but it is
unique, and the implications about the effects of anesthesia are very disquieting; in fact, fully half of the
children exposed to general anesthesia became slow
learners.

The possible impact of general anesthesia is yet another reason why Cesareans should be done only when
absolutely necessary. You should discuss this matter
very carefully with your doctor if he recommends a
Cesarean for you. No mother wants to hear the words
"Your baby is in distress," but usually there is time to
check and recheck this diagnosis—with scalp sampling, a second opinion, and trying natural measures,
such as having the mother change her position, to see
if the baby isn't actually doing fine.

Hypertension: An Exception

Although Cesareans do not generally seem to protect
a baby's neurological development, there may be
groups of babies who are exceptions. The Nassau
County Medical Center on Long Island has taken a
close look at babies who were both underweight and,
for various reasons, delivered before term, usually by
Cesarean. On the whole, these underweight babies did
better on standard tests of neurological and intellectual
skills at ages four and seven the longer they had stayed

in their mothers' wombs; but for a subgroup who were delivered early because their mothers had hypertension, test scores were better the earlier the delivery.

It did not seem to matter whether the mother had chronic hypertension before the pregnancy or whether her high blood pressure was related to "toxemia of pregnancy"; the babies evidently progressed better with nursery care than if they had remained in the uterus of a very sick mother, and, for them, early initiation of labor, even a Cesarean, was beneficial. Much study still needs to be done in this area, however, and it is equally important to note that removing the other sickly or underweight babies early did not seem to help.

Jaundice

Infant jaundice, especially when babies are delivered before spontaneous labor occurs, is another risk that increases with Cesareans. The baby's skin takes on the characteristic yellow color caused by yellow bile, or bilirubin, accumulating in the blood. Most cases of newborn jaundice pass without need for treatment as the baby adjusts to postnatal life. But for some infants, buildups of bilirubin can cause permanent damage, including neurological problems, mental retardation, hearing impairment, incoordination, or psychological disturbances.

Fortunately, in the past decade the treatment of newborn jaundice has improved tremendously. Whereas in the past, badly jaundiced babies had to be transfused, treatment today is usually quite simple: babies are given early, frequent feedings and phototherapy, or exposure to powerful light. Since light causes the bilirubin to break down, in some cases it may be sufficient for the mother to see that the baby receives extra sunlight; other times, the baby has to stay in the hospital until the jaundice disappears. Improved treatment or no, the added days in the hospital upset parents, are costly all around, and make jaundice yet another unnecessary risk of unnecessary Cesareans.

An Experiment with Babies

Finally, because of the great gaps in research on Cesarean section, and especially the absence of long-term follow-up, Cesareans are still an experiment whose consequences cannot be foretold. The increased sophistication of medicine in the post–World War II period has again and again led doctors to think they can "improve" natural pregnancy and labor. Yet intervention in the normal processes of pregnancy has frequently had unexpected unpleasant side effects. We don't have to look far for examples. The synthetic hormone diethylstilbestrol (DES) was lauded as being able to prevent miscarriage and premature birth, and even to ensure "bigger, healthier" babies. About 500,000 to 3 million American mothers took DES until it was learned in 1971 that some daughters of women who took DES during pregnancy were developing rare genital cancers twenty and even thirty years after their birth. Although the cancer rate of DES offspring has, so far, been low, time has also shown that DES children have other problems. The reproductive-tract abnormalities of many daughters make it difficult for them to carry an infant to term, and perhaps 20 percent of DES sons have such low sperm counts that their fertility is doubtful.

As recently as 1976, 10 percent of births in the United States were being artificially induced—usually with hormones—before labor started spontaneously. The arguments for this practice were chillingly similar to the arguments for Cesarean section now: controlled births were "safer" for babies, and scheduling births at times when the hospital had a full staff on hand would enhance survival. Inductions, however, caused respiratory disease and deaths, and launched an epidemic of life-threatening infant jaundice whose aftermath will probably never be fully understood. Since transfusion was then the only treatment for severe jaundice, doctors hesitated to intervene, with the result that thousands of babies were left with neurological deficits, hearing impairments, and other irreparable damage.

Cesareans have already provided one nasty surprise in infant deaths from respiratory disease after repeat operations. We know something about the dangers of inhalation anesthesia, but a lot less than we should know. Is persistent fetal circulation really a Cesarean effect? How seriously does surgery disrupt bonding? What else will we learn, too late? It is so important for you to ask questions, select hospitals and medical personnel carefully, and be informed. Then if you do have to have a Cesarean, you can be confident that the decision was necessary.

Chapter Five

BEING PREPARED FOR SURGERY

When Phyllis Haserot, a New York marketing specialist, went to the hospital to have her first baby, Zane, now three and a half years old, she could hardly believe how easy the birth appeared to be. "I was four centimeters dilated and I hadn't felt a pain yet. The doctor would say, 'You're having a contraction—did you feel it?' And I'd just smile and say, 'No.' We were joking about how I'd probably get through the whole thing without feeling anything, when, one minute later, the baby's heartbeat dropped."

From the sudden drop, the doctor suspected that the umbilical cord was wrapped around the baby's neck— which turned out to be the case—and minutes after the relaxed joking about her easy birth, Phyllis Haserot was having a Cesarean section, under general anesthesia. Because the doctor had to act quickly, there was not enough time for a regional anesthetic, which takes longer to administer. "The worst part, of course, was not being awake and that my husband, Robert, who had been looking forward to the delivery so much, couldn't be there. The next morning, when I really realized what had happened, I just felt sad and cried, but I got over that pretty quickly. At that point, I was very glad I had stayed at my prepared childbirth class when there was a film about Cesareans—I think probably half the class walked out. They weren't interested. Having never been to a hospital for anything, it made me squeamish to watch the blood and surgery at the time, but afterward it gave me some reassurance that I knew what had happened. I do think it's wonderful now that you can learn so much about birth; when you think, barely a decade ago, how unprepared women were, how they weren't taught what to expect at all, it's such an important change."

Education: A Must

Phyllis Haserot is convinced that one reason she recovered quickly from the disappointment of having had a Cesarean was that she had learned about the essentials of the operation ahead of time, even though there was no reason to believe she would not have a normal labor. Yet one of the most difficult issues facing childbirth educators today is how to educate women properly about Cesarean surgery. It is a double bind. On the one hand, we don't want to make Cesareans so terrifying that women who need them are tense and uncooperative, and on the other, there is the danger of making mothers complacent about surgery and muting healthy resistance to Cesareans.

Nancy Cohen, co-founder of C-Sec, Inc., which has led efforts to "humanize" Cesarean section, recalls her own ambivalence about the success of her organization. "What we wanted were things like having fathers allowed at Cesarean deliveries, rooming-in for the babies, and to encourage regional anesthesia so the mother would be awake. A decade ago no one even talked about Cesarean section or how to help the parents through the experience, so we were filling an enormous gap. Within just a few weeks of starting we received hundreds of letters. But, you know, emotionally I had already left the organization within three months. What I really wanted to do was to encourage women *not* to have Cesareans and particularly to work with mothers who had already had a Cesarean, to get them away from automatic repeats and to talk convincingly about V-BAC. It took about three more years for that information to start coming in and when it did I felt it was an incredible disservice for me not to spend all my available time alerting women to the dangers of surgery over V-BAC; and so I left C-Sec."

Whatever their focus, childbirth educators agree that education makes a crucial difference in how a Cesarean affects mothers. If you have a pretty good idea that your prospects for surgery are higher than average—if you are a previous Cesarean mother, diabetic, hypertensive, expecting a breech baby or twins, and so on—you will naturally want to know all you can about the operation. But even if you have none of these problems, with today's Cesarean rate what it is, you would be wise to familiarize yourself with both the details of the operation and ways to make it safer and less painful. Karen Lynch, a New Jersey mother who describes her own Cesarean as "horrible" and is now writing a book on emotional reactions to Cesarean section, has corresponded with dozens of Cesarean mothers. "What has impressed me so far," she comments, "is the range of reactions. It goes from women who had a nervous breakdown afterward to those who were quite satisfied and even happy. And so far, it appears to me that the element which made the most difference is whether the mother was educated about Cesareans. Those who knew nothing usually had the worst time."

First, in learning about Cesarean birth, you will simply need to take many of the same steps and ask many of the same questions as you would when interviewing physicians and investigating hospital policies toward normal birth. For instance, issues like hospital cooperation, "rooming-in" of the infant, and having the baby's father in the delivery room are usually just as important to Cesarean parents as to other parents. If you have a regional anesthetic, the father will be able to support and comfort you and watch his baby being born. "The most important aspect of shared Cesareans is the support that the father can give the mother during the surgery," Christine Wilson and Wendy Hovey write in *Cesarean Childbirth*. "No matter how prepared the mother is, everyone feels some nervousness when a surgical birth is necessary. But the presence of the father can be the single element that makes the difference between the mother feeling confident or anxious at the time of birth. The issue of how the mother feels during birth is not simply a matter of luxury. Extreme anxiety can interfere with the procedure."

Even if you have a general anesthetic, it may be important to have your husband with you. He will be able to tell you about the birth and help you resolve any strangeness or emotional loss you feel about having "missed" your baby's birth. Not all hospitals will allow fathers to be present during Cesareans; also, some fathers, no matter how much they wish to help the mother in every way, may worry that being present for the surgery will make them queasy. While it is very rare for a father to feel sick during a Cesarean—usually fathers get so caught up in the excitement of the birth that they stop really noticing the surgery itself—this is an area where people have to both be frank and respect the choices of others. One Cesarean father, for example, purposely left off his glasses so that he could be there for the benefit of his wife, but still not watch closely. Once again, having a helpful doctor and hospital personnel at hand to discuss these issues will help ensure that everyone comes to comfortable decisions.

Similarly, you may want to have the baby in your room, rather than in the nursery, as soon as you feel well enough. Almost all hospitals now have such rooming-in facilities. If you have a Cesarean with a regional anesthetic, a time period for "bonding" right after the birth may be especially satisfying. Moreover, if you plan to breast-feed, the period after surgery, before the anesthesia wears off and the pain sets in, is an excellent time for the baby's first feeding. So check with your hospital to see what its policies are. Some still require all Cesarean babies—not just those who are ill—to be whisked off to the nursery immediately for observation, but you may find one that appreciates the importance of spending those first moments together. But, beyond issues like these, which are important in all births, you will want to know more specifics about Cesareans.

The Little Things Do Count

Childbirth educators will teach you a lot about vaginal births—what happens when the amniotic sac breaks, about enemas, and so on—but too often they fail to discuss Cesareans in any depth.

"Overall information about Cesareans should be incorporated into childbirth education classes," comments Beth Shearer, a co-founder of C-Sec, Inc., and now its director of information services. "It shouldn't be just a separate topic. It should be discussed with all the other interventions—I mean, one thing so often leads to another—and also discussion of the operation itself should be incorporated with solid information about the necessary, and unnecessary, reasons for it. That way, the women who really do have to have Cesarean sections won't feel cheated by their childbirth educator and ripped off by their doctors. What surprises women most about Cesareans? I would say the biggest surprise is the amount of pain afterward and the slowness of recovery. Mothers get the impression that at least they'll get an anesthetic and get the pain over and the birth out of the way, but it's not quite like that. It can be a real letdown to try to get to know a baby while you're recovering from surgery."

If you know the basic facts beforehand—even the ones that seem unimportant—the surgery will be much less stressful. For example, the sterile solution used to wash your abdomen before the incision usually feels very cold. In some hospitals the pubic hair is shaved completely before the operation, whereas in others only the top inch or two is removed. The less you are shaved, of course, the less itching you will have as the hair grows back. Although most mothers now receive a low horizontal incision, it is important to make sure that any deviation from that is for a good medical reason. "This is much more than a cosmetic request," Beth Shearer explains. "You will be more comfortable in the postpartum period because, with a vertical incision, the baby is always sitting on it when you try to nurse or handle her."

In the postpartum period you will feel some general fatigue and soreness around the incision, but perhaps the greatest physical problem will be the severe gas pains which follow Cesareans and any kind of abdominal surgery. The stress of the surgery on the body causes a loss of potassium in the muscles. Because the body needs potassium to activate enzymes involved in muscle contraction, the potassium depletion may cause the intestinal walls to become partially paralyzed for a few days. When this happens, normal intestinal bacteria ferment and multiply and you have a lot of gas. It might be a good idea to ask your doctor about increasing your potassium intake before surgery. Your body needs about 4,000 milligrams of potassium daily. Such foods as fish, squash, lentils, spinach, and potatoes are good potassium sources. A cup of one of these foods will supply 500 mg or more of potassium. Also, potassium chloride salt, a common substitute for sodium chloride, is available at health-food stores and many supermarkets and supplies about 450 mg per quarter-teaspoon. You can sprinkle it on food or dissolve it in a glass of water. Ask your doctor whether you might take a couple of glasses of water with dissolved potassium as soon as possible after surgery to minimize potassium depletion. However, most doctors have no training in nutrition, so don't be surprised if your doctor doesn't know what to tell you about this.

Sources of Information

With all you are doing to prepare for your baby—learning about normal deliveries and child care, taking classes, getting the baby's room ready—your "study" of Cesareans need not take a long time. The point is to learn the basics—that is, to learn enough to protect yourself. If your childbirth education class does not already include any substantial information about Cesareans, you might ask the instructor to cover basic facts about Cesareans. If she is unprepared, check whether the hospital you have chosen, or another local hospital, routinely shows a film or slide presentation about Cesareans; many hospitals do have "Cesarean shows" separate from routine childbirth education classes, and some even offer special classes for mothers likely to have Cesareans. Your doctor may have a pamphlet about Cesareans available, or you can send away to a Cesarean support group for an information package (see Appendix for list). Also, check your library or bookstore for the several books now available on the subject.

Choosing Anesthesia

Anesthesia is a special concern for Cesarean parents. It is important that you have a working knowledge of the pros and cons of general and regional anesthesia so that you can discuss them with your doctor and make decisions confidently. Most mothers will probably want a regional unless an emergency or special circumstances necessitate a general anesthetic. On the other hand, just as there are fathers who really do not want to be present for a Cesarean, there are also mothers who find the whole prospect of surgery so overwhelming that they want to be put to sleep. It is your choice, but before you reject the safer regional, remember that your abdomen can be screened during the delivery, so you can have the advantages of a regional without actually having to see anything.

The regionals used for Cesareans are primarily epidurals and spinals. There are sometimes medical reasons for choosing one or the other, but most women prefer an epidural because it is less painful to administer and permits more movement. With either, you will feel numb from about the waist down, but you may feel some pulling and tugging as the baby is removed. As long as you are prepared for this, it should not be alarming, and will help you feel that you are participating in your baby's birth.

Often doctors will give mothers a sedative or tranquilizer to relax them before administering the regional. You don't have to take it, however. It will make you sleepy and interfere with your alertness for your baby's birth. When Julia Houston, a Brooklyn mother, went for her second Cesarean, one of her major decisions about confronting the operation differently was not to be sedated. "I was very naïve the first time," she recalls. "I had Demerol and all sorts of things and felt horrible. What I wanted the second time was to be as much in control of the birth as I could. The doctors teased me sometimes. They kept saying, 'Oh, here comes the one who doesn't want to be sedated.' But what I really wanted was to be absolutely myself during the birth and not some groggy package messenger delivering a baby. It made all the difference. When the baby appeared and I was really awake, that was what I wanted."

Also, some doctors routinely put out the mother for the surgical repair after the birth. There is rarely any medical need for this, and it eliminates the possibility of your spending those important first minutes with your new baby. Talk all these things over with your doctor, and with the anesthesiologist, so that you all understand each other's wishes before the operation begins.

Finally, even though it is unlikely that you will find an obstetrician who uses local anesthesia—and in some areas of the country, it is still hard for women to find hospitals where regionals are readily available—you may want to at least inquire about this. The procedure may seem a little daunting—the mother usually has twelve shots of Novocain in the abdomen—but is actually faster to administer than a spinal or epidural and probably no more painful. The great advantage is its safety to both the mother and child. In fact, for mothers who have heart conditions or other serious illnesses which make it dangerous for them to have anesthesia, the safety of locals is really important—as it is for babies who are extremely sick or distressed. "I can tell you that the happiest person when we switched to local anesthesia was our pediatrician," comments Dr. Ranney, an absolute believer in the locals for Cesareans. "I've seen very premature, two-pound infants come out kicking and crying with a local, whereas with a general, you would have had to spend a half hour resuscitating them. The other beauty of this technique is that you can teach it to an intern in about two births and then he'll know about as much about it as I do. You've given him a safe method of anesthesia for Cesareans that he can use in an emergency or set up in a desert if he has to."

To Try Labor or Not

Mothers who expect beforehand that they have a high prospect for a Cesarean—those who have already had one Cesarean, those with an unturned breech, and so on—will want to discuss carefully the advantages of going into labor before the surgery. Obviously, waiting for the spontaneous start of labor, rather than scheduling the operation, helps protect the baby from respiratory distress syndrome. But there may be medical reasons for a scheduled operation. If the mother lives in a small community where there is no hospital that has an operating room open twenty-four hours a day, the doctor may not want to risk having to rouse the staff into action at the last minute.

Psychological Support

If you have just had a Cesarean, especially an unexpected one, it is quite natural for you to feel upset. Anger, depression, confusion, and guilt at "failing" to have a normal birth are all common after a Cesarean. Your husband may not fully understand your emotions, and your doctor may find it difficult to discuss your feelings because some of the anger is likely to be directed at him. "How often I have heard women say how angry they were for months after a Cesarean section—angry at their doctors for violating their bodies, angry at their baby for having been there and making them go through this the way they did, and angry at themselves for having failed at a basic biological function," Dr. Richard Hausknecht, an obstetrician at the Mt. Sinai School of Medicine in New York, has written. "I think most physicians, and I include myself in this, are astonished to hear some of the feelings that come up, because we tend not to want to hear it."

But if you look for support from people who know exactly what you've been through, you may find that their assistance is invaluable. A nurse or your childbirth educator may be able to put you in contact with a local Cesarean support group—they now exist in hundreds of American communities—or just look in the phone book. Talking about your feelings with women who have had the same experience—and the same wrenching emotions—can be enormously constructive. Also, even though your husband or friends may not fully understand your complex feelings at this time, they can still help with child care and housework, and in other ways that are cheering. Remember that postsurgical physical exhaustion can contribute to depression, so look for help to combat that exhaustion. One mother remembers her delight when, just before going for her second Cesarean, she read her insurance policy very carefully and realized the policy would cover the costs of a private nurse while she was still in the hospital. "What a difference that made," she says. "I always got my painkillers right on time and the nurse gave me frequent sponge baths. Does that ever give you a boost when you're feeling grubby after surgery."

Perhaps most immediately helpful, if you learned nothing about Cesareans in advance or had an entirely unexpected operation, is to have your doctor, a nurse, or a childbirth educator explain exactly what went on during your operation and what made it necessary. Some Cesarean mothers even find it useful to attend Cesarean classes after the birth. In this vein, Gail Winston, an editor, recalls that her doctor helped her a great deal in coming to terms with her unexpected Cesarean. "He bent over backward the next morning to explain the reasons to me," she says, "and I have to say it never seemed like a big, horrible thing to me; I was convinced it was correct for that birth—although next time I want to try a normal birth. I suppose the worst problem is when you think the wrong decision has been made, but that's not what I thought. I began to think I would end up with a Cesarean hours before they even suggested it."

As their physical strength returns and they start taking care of their infant, most mothers find great delight in the baby. Yet, it is still not unusual for mothers to have lingering depressions which they can hardly explain themselves. If this is your experience, think over all the things that might be bothering you. One mother, for example, recalls her fury at waking up from general anesthesia, feeling absolutely terrible, to find her husband making phone calls to relatives and generally acting like a new father when she herself did not truly feel like a new mother. As it turned out—months later, when they finally discussed it—he had also been quite angry about the Cesarean and upset not to have been allowed into the operating room for his child's birth, but thought he should disguise his own disappointment for his wife's sake. As she realized her husband's true concerns, she felt a lot better—and better understood.

Or, Esther Zorn suggests, if you feel that the Cesarean is interfering with your relations with your infant, or keeps making you angrier than it is comfortable to be, try psychotherapy if that's what is needed. "We are," she adds, "all Cesarean mothers first and we still feel the frustration, but we also have to learn to go on."

Once again, however, with preparation, you can lessen the emotional and physical shock of a Cesarean; you can have a sense of control over your baby's birth —a sense that you are making it the satisfying occasion it should be.

————————AFTERWORD————————

The Social Costs of Cesarean Section

While the medical risks of Cesarean section must be our first concern, we cannot ignore the social costs of Cesareans—particularly the financial aspects of delivering almost 20 percent of American babies by surgery. Cesareans cost a great deal of money; at an average of about $4,000 each, America's 600,000 annual Cesareans now consume about $2.5 billion in health-care dollars. The 1979 University of Washington study which focused on repeat mothers alone concluded that, for every 10,000 previous Cesarean mothers who tried labor, even if some ended up having another section, there was a saving of $5 million for surgery and hospital charges alone, and another $1.2 million saved for fetal maturity tests which didn't have to be done. This total of more than $6 million, calculated in 1979, would now be about $10 to $12 million for every 10,000 trial labors—or a national saving of $100 to $120 million if even half of today's 200,000 annual automatic repeat mothers were encouraged to labor.

When you start talking about millions and billions in health-care dollars, you must look closely at both the personal and the public impact. For parents, the cost of a Cesarean is often devastating. Physicians' fees are usually about double that for vaginal birth, as are hospital costs. In Manhattan, where a few years ago the *New York Times* estimated that average obstetricians' fees for Cesarean deliveries ranged between $3,000 and $4,500, average reimbursement to parents individually insured under the most popular Blue Shield plan was only $300. Parents had to pay the difference themselves. Company or union-sponsored insurance plans may pay more than individual ones, but even the best plans will leave parents to pay a good chunk of the obstetrician's fee. "I don't mean to complain," says one father, whose three children under age five were all Cesarean babies delivered at Southampton Hospital, which holds the dubious distinction of having the highest Cesarean rate in New York State. "But you can really feel the burden. It is just a lot of money."

Aside from the financial strain on parents, it is an equal disgrace that such huge amounts of money should be diverted from measures which could truly enhance the health of children. In the United States, where perinatal survival lags behind much of the Western world—and behind such places as Singapore and Hong Kong—probably nothing would more benefit infant health than to concentrate on good prenatal care, and especially on preventing prematurity, with its high risk of both infant deaths and lifelong disabilities. For instance, we know that when women smoke more than a pack of cigarettes a day during pregnancy, the rate of prematurity among their babies doubles. Yet there is probably not a single hospital in the United States which offers a smoking-cessation program as a routine part of its prenatal care, and there are no public programs at all to assist pregnant women to stop smoking.

The experience at New York Hospital, where diabetic mothers who had excellent, intensive prenatal care and were well instructed in nutrition delivered healthier babies than the average clinic mother—and New York Hospital does not even see the concentration of sickly and neglected mothers routine for slum hospitals—is a profound reproach to standard prenatal care in the United States. Would anything more improve American infant health and survival than to take half the budget for unnecessary Cesareans and use it to subsidize prenatal care and nutrition? The Women's, Infant's and Children's Program of the Department of Agriculture is now the only national program which supplies food and nutritional advice to pregnant mothers; its success in reducing the numbers of premature and underweight infants is well documented. However, funded to serve fewer than one million pregnancies a year, the program cannot take all mothers who want and need its services. Even as unnecessary Cesareans mount, the United States continues to pay for its neglect of pregnancy care in its lagging infant survival.

On Lawsuits

Obstetricians are sued for malpractice ten times more often than other doctors. They are sued if they do Cesareans and if they don't. They are sued if there is anything wrong with the baby—even in obvious cases of genetic malformation. In a recent California case, a mother sued over an infection that developed after a Cesarean which was performed because she had visible herpes lesions at the time of delivery; in this case, there was no choice about surgery and, as we have seen, it is impossible to guard against all infection after Cesareans, even when the mother is given prophylactic antibiotics.

Every parent must be concerned about the strains and distortions which legal suits have placed on the practice of obstetrics. If you are considering a legal action against your doctor after childbirth, I urge you to think carefully about what you are doing. If parents seriously think that the conduct of the birth process permanently injured either the baby or the mother, that is one matter. If you are suing because you are angry— even justifiably—or upset about the birth, or were somehow inconvenienced, or for a minor injury that heals quickly, that is another question altogether.

Even if you had a Cesarean that you are now absolutely certain was unnecessary, a legal suit will never change the method of birth or "give you back" a normal delivery. Quite the contrary, as long as you are focused on a legal suit, you will also be focused on what was "wrong" about the birth, rather than on what is right about your new baby. Legal suits often last for years, they place a considerable strain on parents, and despite the publicity given to those who win large settlements, their outcome is uncertain. At the least, any parents thinking of starting a legal suit owe it to themselves to go to a medical library and read a 1977 article called "Litigation Produced Pain, Disease and Suffering," by Dr. Robert Brent in the journal *Teratology;* it will give them considerable insight into some of the strains they may face.

But most important for parents concerned about unnecessary Cesareans, lawsuits have done nothing to curb the Cesarean explosion; they are in fact a major contributing factor to it. This does not mean, however, that there are no actions you can take if you feel you have been subjected to an unnecessary Cesarean. There are other—and more effective—arenas than court. You can make detailed, written complaints to the administration of the hospital, its chairman of obstetrics, the local and state health departments, and to the professional society regulating obstetricians in your area. You will not, of course, always receive courteous attention when you do this; you will not always be satisfied that your complaint has been well investigated. However, in the end, the doctor will feel more pressure to rethink his Cesarean decisions than if he was sued. If he is a true incompetent—and particularly if there have been other complaints about him—it is possible he will lose his license or, at the least, his privileges to practice at his hospital. If your desire is to enhance the practice of obstetrics in this country, your complaints to health officials will ultimately have more impact than a lawsuit.

—————————————APPENDIX—————————————

Major Organizations for Birth Information

The following organizations distribute a variety of publications on childbirth, and are especially interested in the problem of Cesareans. From among them you should be able to obtain good advice about any special problems or questions you may have. The best procedure is usually to send first for the organization's publication list. Include a large self-addressed stamped envelope, and a donation of a dollar or two to cover the cost of sending you the list. These organizations are run largely by volunteers; they will later charge you a minimal fee for any special books or publications you order.

C-Sec, Inc.
22 Forest Road
Framingham, MA 01701
(617) 877-8266

International Childbirth Education Association (ICEA)
P.O. Box 20048
Minneapolis, MN 55420
(612) 854-8660

Maternity Center Association
48 East 92nd Street
New York, NY 10028
(212) 369-7300

National Association of Parents and Professionals
  for Safe Alternatives in Childbirth
P.O. Box 267
Marble Hill, MO 63764
(314) 238-2010

Cesarean Prevention Movement, Inc.
P.O. Box 152, University Station
Syracuse, NY 13210
(315) 424-1942

Cesarean Prevention Movement:
 Directory of Chapters

Main Office:
  Cesarean Prevention Movement, Inc.
  P.O. Box 152
  Syracuse, NY 13210
  National President: Esther Booth Zorn
  315-424-1942

Regional Directors:

  Northeast: Jan Griffin
  140-30 Alcott Pl.
  Bronx, NY 10475
  212-379-4716

  South: Justine Clegg
  5520 S.W. 92 Ave.
  Miami, FL 33165
  305-596-2699

  Midwest: Barbara Hotze
  810 Haymount Dr.
  Indianapolis, IN 46241
  317-243-9616

  West: Dee Ottero
  505 North 25th
  Grand Junction, CO 81501
  303-243-7450

Canada/Overseas:
Marianne Brorup-Weston
2127-A Hemlock St. RR #2
Terrace, British Columbia,
Canada V86 3Z9
604-635-2942

Local Chapters:
CPM of Central New York
1008 Westcott St.
Syracuse, NY 13210
Contact Person: Esther Zorn
315-424-1942

CPM of North Jersey, New Jersey
2 Walnut Circle
Basking Ridge, NJ 07920
Contact Person: Ruth Lufkin
201-766-0311

CPM of Gloucester, Massachusetts
Hillside Rd.
Gloucester, MA 01930
Contact Person: Ellen Hedendal
617-283-0520

CPM of Lafayette, Indiana
909 N. Wagon Wheel Trail
Lafayette, IN 47905
Contact Person: Susan Hess
317-474-8194

CPM of Indianapolis, Indiana
4143 E. 61st St.
Indianapolis, IN 46220
Contact Person: Jane Warren
317-253-5634

CPM of Western Indiana
RR 5 Box 493B
Terre Haute, IN 47805
Contact Person: Amy Papinchock

CPM of Sacramento, California
8280 Woodman Ln.
Newcastle, CA 95658
Contact Person: Tece Markel
916-362-9739

CPM of Wichita, Kansas
P.O. Box 18363
Wichita, KS 67218
Contact Person: Kris Berger
316-265-0237

CPM of Brandermill, VA
1400 Whispering Oaks Rd.
Midlothian, VA 23113
Contact Person: Karen Halvorson, RN

CPM of Madison, Wisconsin
1416 E. Dayton
Madison, WI 53703
Contact Person: Mary Jo Schiavoni
608-255-6931

CPM of Southeast Michigan
904 N. Rembrandt
Royal Oak, MI 48067
Contact Person: Janice Frasher McIntosh
313-548-8033

CPM of Toronto, Ontario, Canada
c/o 42 Roseheath Ave.
Toronto, Ontario
Canada M4J 3E8
Contact Person: Valerie Christenson
416-690-3901

The Five Centers for Home Treatment of Diabetes During Pregnancy

Andrea Fischl, M.P.H.
Diabetes Research Center

Iroquois Building, Suite 502
3600 Forbes Avenue
Pittsburgh, PA 15213
Phone (412) 647-5200

Barbara Plovie, R.N.
University of Washington at Seattle
571 Harborview Hall ZA-36
326 9th Avenue
Seattle, WA 98104
Phone (206) 223-3046

Anne Dukles, R.N.
Diabetes and Pregnancy
334 East 63rd Street
New York, NY 10021
Phone (212) 838-4402

Chris Wasson, R.N.
Diabetes and Early Pregnancy Program
Seeley Mudd Building
250 Longwood Avenue
Boston, MA 02115
Phone (617) 732-2006

Dr. Carole Ober, Ph.D.
Prentice Women's Hospital—Maternity Center
Northwestern Memorial Hospital
333 East Superior Street
Chicago, IL 60611
Phone (312) 649-6478

NOTES

The following notes, which are arranged by page according to chapter, cite the major studies referred to in the text. Virtually all direct quotes not otherwise identified have come from personal or telephone interviews.

Chapter One

page
19   Minkoff, H., and R. Schwartz, "The Rising Cesarean Section Rate: Can It Safely Be Reversed?" *Obstetrics and Gynecology* 56:135–43, 1980.

Haverkamp, A., et al., "Differential Effects of Intrapartum Fetal Monitoring," *American Journal of Obstetrics and Gynecology* 134:399–408, 1979.

Kolata, G., "NIH Panel Urges Fewer Cesarean Births," *Science* 210:176–77, 1980.

23   Marieskind, H., *An Evaluation of Cesarean Section in the United States* (Washington, D.C.: Department of Health, Education and Welfare, 1979), "Physiological Costs to Mother," pp. 43–55.

24   Ibid., "Physiological Costs to Infant," pp. 55–60.

26   Baird, Sir D., "Caesarean Section: Its Use in Difficult Labor in Primagravidae," *British Medical Journal* 2:1159, 1955.

O'Driscoll, K., and M. Foley, "Cesarean Birth and Perinatal Mortality," *Obstetrics and Gynecology* 61:1–5, 1983.

33   Shy, K., et al., "Evaluation of Repeat Cesarean Section
      as a Standard of Care: An Application of Decision
      Analysis," *American Journal of Obstetrics and
      Gynecology* 139:123–29, 1981.
36   "Summary Statement," National Institutes of Health
      Consensus Development Conference, Vol. 3, No. 6.
      (Washington, D.C.: U.S. Government Printing Of-
      fice, 1980), p. 1.
38   Marieskind, op. cit., pp. 82–87.
39   Norwood, C., "A Relatively Low Cesarean Rate in an
      Urban Population: Lessons from the New York City
      Municipal Hospital System." Unpublished study,
      1981. Summarized in *New York Times,* December
      15, 1981, p. C6.
41   "Summary Statement, op. cit., p. 2.
43   Barton, J., et al., "The Efficacy of X-ray Pelvimetry,"
      American Journal of Obstetrics and Gynecology
      143:304–11, 1982.
      Jagani, N., et. al., "The Predictability of Labor Out-
      come from a Comparison of Birth Weight and X-ray
      Pelvimetry," *American Journal of Obstetrics and
      Gynecology* 139:507–11, 1981.
46   Haverkamp et al., op. cit.
48   Goodlin, R., "Low-Risk Obstetric Care for Low-Risk
      Mothers," *Lancet,* May 10, 1980, pp. 1017–19.
49   Haesslein, H., and K. Niswander, "Fetal Distress in
      Term Pregnancies," *American Journal of Obstetrics
      and Gynecology* 137:245, 1980.
53   Ranney, B., "The Gentle Art of External Cephalic Ver-
      sion," *American Journal of Obstetrics and Gynecol-
      ogy* 116:239–51, 1973.

Chapter Two

page
63   Norwood, C., "Cesarean Surgery? You Decide." *New
      York Daily News,* August 22, 1982, p. 21.
67   Francome, C., and P. Huntingford, "Births by Caesar-
      ean Section in the United States of America and in

Britain," *Journal of Biosocial Science* 12:353–62, 1980.

68   Sack, R., "The Effect of Utilization on Health Care Costs," *American Journal of Obstetrics and Gynecology* 137:271–73, 1980.

Bean, Constance, *Methods of Childbirth* (New York: Dolphin Books, 1982), p. 216.

76   Maisels, M., et al., "Elective Delivery of the Term Fetus: An Obstetrical Hazard," *Journal of the American Medical Association* 238:2036–38, 1977.

77   Monheit, A., and L. Cousins, "When Do You Measure Scalpblood pH?" *Contemporary Obstetrics and Gynecology* 18:107–21, 1981.

80   Norwood, C., "Delivering Babies the Old-Fashioned Way," *New York Magazine,* August 25, 1982, p. 66.

83   Bennetts, A., and R. Lubic, "The Free-Standing Birth Centre," *Lancet,* February 13, 1982, pp. 378–80.

86   Friedman, E., and M. Sachtleben, "Station of the Fetal Presenting Part," *Obstetrics and Gynecology* 36:558–67, 1970.

87   Flynn, A., et al., "Ambulation in Labor," *British Medical Journal,* August 26, 1978, pp. 591–93.

89   Hughey, M., et al., "Maternal and Fetal Outcome of Lamaze-Prepared Patients," *Obstetrics and Gynecology* 51:643–47, 1978.

92   Taylor, P., in discussion following H. Hopwood, "Shoulder Dystocia: Fifteen Years' Experience in a Community Hospital," *American Journal of Obstetrics and Gynecology* 144:162–66, 1982.

Turner, G., and E. Collins, "Maternal Effects: Fetal Effects of Regular Salicylate Ingestion in Pregnancy," *Lancet,* August 23, 1975, pp. 335–39.

93   Sokol, R., et al., "Computer Diagnosis of Labor Progression," *American Journal of Obstetrics and Gynecology* 119:767–74, 1974.

94   Bean, op. cit., p. 74.

96   Young, D., and C. Mahan, *Unnecessary Cesareans: Ways to Avoid Them* (Minneapolis: International Childbirth Education Association, 1980), pp. 10–11.

228   NOTES

98   Davis, Adelle, *Let's Eat Right to Keep Fit* (New York: New American Library (Signet), 1970), p. 166.

Chapter Three

page
111 Callen, P., et al., "Mode of Delivery and the Lecithin/ Sphyngomyelin Ratio," *British Journal of Obstetrics and Gynecology* 86:965–68, 1979.
112 Shy, et al., op. cit.
115 Chervenak, F., and H. Shamsi, "Is Amniocentesis Necessary Before Elective Repeat Cesarean Section?" *Obstetrics and Gynecology* 60:305–8, 1982.
116 Saldana, L., et al., "Management of Pregnancy After Cesarean Section," *American Journal of Obstetrics and Gynecology* 135:555–61, 1979.
     Morewood, G., et al., "Vaginal Delivery After Cesarean Section," *Obstetrics and Gynecology* 42:589–95, 1973.
     Gibbs, C., "Planned Vaginal Delivery Following Cesarean Section," *Clinics in Obstetrics and Gynecology* 23:507–15, 1980.
120 Cohen, N., and L. Estner, *Silent Knife: Cesarean Prevention and Vaginal Birth After Cesarean Section* (South Hadley, Mass.: Bergin and Garvey, 1983), p. 112.
121 Demianczuk, N., et al., "Trial of Labor After Previous Cesarean Section," *American Journal of Obstetrics and Gynecology* 142:640–42, 1982.
127 Green, J., et al., "Has an Increased Cesarean Section Rate for Term Breech Delivery Reduced the Incidence of Birth Asphyxia, Trauma, and Death?" *American Journal of Obstetrics and Gynecology* 142:643–48, 1982.
129 Collea, J., et al., "The Randomized Management of Term Frank Breech Presentation," *American Journal of Obstetrics and Gynecology* 137:235–44, 1980.
130 Gimovsky, M., et. al., "Randomized Management of the Non-Frank Breech Presentation at Term: A Preliminary Report," *American Journal of Obstetrics and Gynecology* 146:34–40, 1983.

132 Ranney, op. cit.
136 Van Dorsten, J., et al., "Randomized Control Trial of External Cephalic Version with Tocolysis in Late Pregnancy," *American Journal of Obstetrics and Gynecology* 141:417–24, 1981.
140 Yeh, S., and J. Read, "Management of Post-Term Pregnancy in a Large Obstetric Population," *Obstetrics and Gynecology* 60:282–87, 1982.
142 Freeman, R., et al., "Postdate Pregnancy," *American Journal of Obstetrics and Gynecology* 140:131–33, 1981.

Cohen, op. cit., p. 178.
143 Elliott, J., and J. Flaherty, "The Use of Breast Stimulation to Ripen the Cervix in Term Pregnancies," *American Journal of Obstetrics and Gynecology* 145:553–56, 1983.
144 Sokol, op. cit.
145 Friedman, E., and M. Sachtleben, "Relation of Maternal Age to the Course of Labor," *American Journal of Obstetrics and Gynecology* 91:915–22, 1965.
148 Corey, L., "The Diagnosis and Treatment of Genital Herpes," *Journal of the American Medical Association* 248:1041–49, 1982.
150 Corwin, R., in discussion following L. Vontver et al., "Recurrent Genital Herpes Simplex Virus Infection in Pregnancy," *American Journal of Obstetrics and Gynecology* 143:75–83, 1982.
154 Jovanovic, L., et al., "Effect of Euglycemia on the Outcome of Pregnancy in Insulin-Dependent Diabetic Women," *American Journal of Medicine* 71:921–27, 1981.
156 Coustan, D., et al., "Tight Metabolic Control of Overt Diabetes in Pregnancy," *American Journal of Medicine* 68:845–52, 1980.

Roversi, A., et al., "A New Approach to the Treatment of Diabetic Pregnant Women," *American Journal of Obstetrics and Gynecology* 135:567–76, 1979.

Jovanovic, R., "Term Delivery of the Diabetic Patient." Paper delivered at 10th World Congress of Obstetrics and Gynecology, San Francisco, October 1982.

159   Hawrylyshyn, P., et al., "Twin Pregnancies—A Continuing Perinatal Challenge," *Obstetrics and Gynecology* 59:463–66, 1982.

Kelsick, F., and H. Minkoff, "Management of the Breech Second Twin," *American Journal of Obstetrics and Gynecology* 144:783–86, 1982.

160   Loucopoulos, A., and R. Jewelewicz, "Management of Multifetal Pregnancies," *American Journal of Obstetrics and Gynecology* 143:902–5, 1982.

Chapter Four

page
170   Ranney, B., "The Advantages of Local Anesthesia for Cesarean Section," *Obstetrics and Gynecology* 45:163–67, 1982.

171   Marieskind, op. cit., pp. 45–50.

172   Collea et al., op. cit.

173   Baird, Sir D., op. cit.

174   Meier, G., "Maternal Behaviour of Feral- and Laboratory-Reared Monkeys Following the Surgical Delivery of Their Infants," *Nature* 206:492–93, 1965.

175   Klaus, M., et al., "Maternal Attachment: Importance of the First Post-partum Days," *New England Journal of Medicine* 286:460–63, 1972.

Sugarman, M., "Paranatal Influences on Maternal-Infant Attachment," *American Journal of Orthopsychiatry* 47:407–21, 1977.

178   Minkoff and Schwartz, op. cit.

180   Chervenak and Shamsi, op. cit.

181   Maisels et al., op. cit.

Schreiner, R., et al., "Respiratory Distress Following Elective Repeat Cesarean Section," *American Journal of Obstetrics and Gynecology* 142:689–92, 1982.

183   Ranney, et al., op. cit.

185   Norwood, unpublished study, op. cit.

190   Haverkamp, et al., op. cit.

191   Haesslein and Niswander, op. cit.

Niswander, K., "The Obstetrician, Fetal Asphyxia and Cerebral Palsy," *American Journal of Obstetrics and Gynecology* 133:358–61, 1979.

193 Brackbill, Y., and S. Broman, "Obstetrical Medication and Development in the First Year of Life." (Draft.) Bethesda, Md., National Institute of Neurological and Communicative Disorders and Stroke, January 1979.

Ranney et al., op. cit.

194 Winer, E., N. Tejani, et al., "Four- to Seven-Year Evaluation in Two Groups of Small-for-Gestational Age Infants," *American Journal of Obstetrics and Gynecology* 143:425–29, 1982.

Chapter Five

page
204 Wilson, C., and W. Hovey, *Cesarean Childbirth* (New York: New American Library (Signet), 1981), p. 228.

205 McClellan, M., and W. Cabianca, "Effects of Early Mother-Infant Contact Following Cesarean Birth," *Obstetrics and Gynecology* 56:52–55, 1980.

212 Bowers, S., et. al., "Prevention of Iatrogenic Respiratory Distress Syndrome," *American Journal of Obstetrics and Gynecology*," 143:186–89, 1982.

Hausknecht, R., "The Responsbility of the Physician in Meeting Cesarean Patient and Parent Needs," in *A Humanistic Approach to Cesarean Childbirth* (San Jose, Calif.: Cesarean Birth Council International, 1981), pp. 18–26.

─────SELECTED READINGS─────

Selected readings on avoiding Cesareans or other unnecessary interferences with normal labor:

Arms, Suzanne. *Immaculate Deception.* New York: Bantam Books, 1977.

Cohen, N., and L. Estner. *Silent Knife: Cesarean Prevention and Vaginal Birth After Cesarean* (1983). Available by sending $14.95 plus $1.25 for shipping to Bergin and Garvey Publishers, Inc., 670 Amherst Road, South Hadley, MA 01075.

Young, D., and C. Mahan. *Unnecessary Cesareans: Ways to Avoid Them* (1980). Pamphlet, available for $1.50 plus $1.00 postage from International Childbirth Education Association Bookcenter, P. O. Box 20048, Minneapolis, MN 55420.

Major sources of information about alternatives in childbirth:

NAPSAC Directory of Alternative Birth Services and Consumer Guide, 1982.
   Lists 4,000 birth services in the United States, including alternative birth centers, parent education classes, practicing midwives, and labor coaches.
   Available for $5.95 from National Association of Parents and Professionals for Safe Alternatives in Childbirth, P. O. Box 267, Marble Hill, MO 63764.

The Whole Birth Catalog (1983), J. Ashford, ed.
   A highly comprehensive catalog listing books about childbirth, organizations, and other resources.
   Available for $14.95 plus $1.00 postage from The Crossing Press, Trumansburg, NY 14886.

233

eating and drinking during, 97–98
father's presence during, 204–5
internal examinations during, 99
mother's posture in, 26–27, 50–51, 96, 132, 194
natural encouragement of, 26–27, 51, 87, 96–99, 194
painful, 90, 92, 94–95
parents' roles in, 70, 79, 89–92, 99–100, 131–32
phases of, 86–87, 94, 146
trial, *see* trial labor
see also dystocia
Labor of Love service, 122–23
"labor support" persons, 96, 102–3, 122
La Leche League, 71
Lamaze techniques, 28, 89–90, 163
Lancet, 48, 83
lex caesarea, 21
litigation, *see* malpractice suits
"Litigation Produced Pain, Disease and Suffering" (Brent), 218–19
local anesthesia, 95, 169–70, 183–184, 210–11
Lopez, Antonio, III, 109
Lopez, Miriam, 109
Los Angeles Women's Hospital, 35, 57, 67, 74, 80, 118, 129–30, 139–42
love making, overdue babies and, 142–43
L/S ratio, 180–82
Lubic, Ruth, 36
Lynch, Karen, 203–4

malpractice suits, 38–40, 49, 150–151, 217–19
Cesareans as protection from, 38–40, 125
complaints vs., 219
Marieskind, Helen, 37–39
maternal death rates, 23, 33, 97, 112, 168–69
Maternity Center Association, 36, 82–83
meconium, inhalation of, 187
Medical Forum, 167
menstrual dates, miscalculation of, 139, 142–43
meperidine (Demerol), 93–94, 146, 210

Methods of Childbirth (Bean), 69, 94
midwives, 57, 71, 79–83, 104–5
breech babies and, 130–31
mothers:
anxiety of, 26, 47, 69, 99, 122, 147
health of, 31–32, 66, 110, 144, 147–58, 188, 195, 211
high-risk, *see* high-risk mothers
infants' attachment to, 175–77
minority, 66–67
special instructions of, 73, 77
support for, 122, 161–64, 212–14
see also older mothers
Ms., 51
multiple births, 110, 159–60

National Maternity Hospital (Dublin, Ireland), 95, 178, 185
natural childbirth, 26–28, 51, 79–84, 90–91, 96–100
doctors' views on, 90–91, 100
safety of, 80–83
technological approach vs., 27–28
neonatal deaths, 65–66, 134
Neonatal Intensive Care Unit, Hershey Medical Center, 76–77, 181
neonatal jaundice, 24, 195–97
neurological abnormalities, *see* brain damage
New York Times, 216
nicking amniotic sac membranes, 29
night deliveries, 72–73
nitrous oxide, infants affected by, 193
Nolan, Pat, 163–64
non-stress tests, 140–41, 157
"Normal Birth Center," Los Angeles Women's Hospital, 35
North Central Bronx Hospital, 35, 63, 67, 74, 88, 91, 97, 99, 121
midwife births at, 57, 80–81, 121
Novocain, 170, 183, 210
nurses, private, 102–3, 213
nutrition, 97–99, 207–8, 217
calcium and, 98–99
potassium in, 207–8

Oberlander, Samuel, 120–21
Odent, Michael, 132

ABOUT THE AUTHOR

CHRISTOPHER NORWOOD is a medical-environmental journalist who from 1980 to 1981 was Communications Director of the New York City Health and Hospitals Corporation. Her most recent book, *At Highest Risk: Environmental Hazards to Young and Unborn Children*, was a *Library Journal* selection as one of the best medical science books of 1980. Her earlier book, *About Paterson: The Making and Unmaking of an American City*, was selected by *The New York Times* as a "Significant Book of the Year" in 1974.